REVERSE AGING WITH PEPTIDES

Unlocking Youthful Vitality and Health through Cutting-Edge Science

Lois Mcgrath MD

All rights reserved. No part of this publication may be reproduced, distributed, or transmitted in any form or by any means, including photocopying, recording, or other electronic or mechanical methods, without the prior written permission of the publisher, except in the case of brief quotations embodied in critical reviews and certain other noncommercial uses permitted by copyright law.

Copyright © Lois mcgrath, 2024.

Table of contents

INTRODUCTION

At sixty-two, Karen felt her body was aging faster than she was ready to accept. She loved spending time with her grandchildren, hiking trails, and staying active, but more often than not, her body seemed to disagree. Each year brought new signs of age—aching joints, slower recovery after exercise, and the inevitable appearance of wrinkles and thinning hair. Even her energy, once boundless, seemed to diminish with every passing season. For a woman who had always valued her health and vitality, these changes were not just disappointing—they were disheartening.

A visit to a holistic health clinic in search of guidance would change everything. There, Karen learned about peptides and how they were being used to support the body's natural repair processes, essentially helping people age more gracefully. The practitioner explained that peptides were like specialized tools designed to target specific parts of the body—helping the skin retain elasticity, encouraging muscles to recover faster, and even supporting energy levels. Karen was intrigued but cautious. She'd tried countless creams, supplements, and regimens over the years, only to be disappointed. Yet, something about this concept seemed different.

After a detailed consultation, she decided to start a carefully monitored peptide program. Within weeks, Karen noticed subtle changes: her joints felt less achy, her energy was on the rise, and even her skin had a healthier glow. Months into the routine, she found herself moving with the ease she'd had a decade earlier. Her confidence grew as she saw visible changes that matched how she felt inside—vibrant, resilient, and ready to embrace life fully.

Karen's story isn't unique. She represents thousands of people discovering a new approach to aging that doesn't involve invasive procedures, high-risk medications, or empty promises. Instead, it's rooted in the power of peptides—a tool the body can recognize and put to use. Welcome to a new era of anti-aging, where we're no longer limited by time but instead empowered by science.

A New Era of Anti-Aging

The desire to age gracefully is universal, but traditional methods of anti-aging have often left people disappointed or even skeptical. For years, the marketplace has offered products that promise youth in a jar, promising miraculous results without sufficient science to back them up. This approach has made many people wary, creating a sense of resignation that aging is something we just have to accept. But recent advancements have opened doors that, until recently, were only speculative.

In today's world, we're standing at the forefront of a revolutionary approach to health, where anti-aging isn't about defying nature but about aligning with it. Scientific research has now highlighted ways to support the body in maintaining its vitality well into advanced years. Peptides represent one of the most exciting frontiers in this area—these small chains of amino acids are already naturally present in our bodies and perform crucial functions, from aiding muscle recovery to supporting skin regeneration.

Imagine feeling more energetic, seeing smoother skin, and enjoying increased flexibility, all from substances that work harmoniously with the body. This isn't wishful thinking; it's the essence of what peptides bring to the table. By integrating peptides into our health routines, we are not introducing foreign elements but rather enhancing what the body already knows how to do—repair, regenerate, and thrive.

The Power of Peptides in Rejuvenation

Peptides are often described as the building blocks of proteins, but they are much more than that. They are signaling agents, communicators that tell cells what to do and when. When we age, the natural production of peptides in the body declines, and with it, so does our ability to repair and regenerate. Wrinkles, joint stiffness, slower muscle recovery, and fatigue are common indicators of this decline.

What makes peptides so compelling in the field of anti-aging is their specificity. Each peptide type has a unique role, targeting specific issues with precision that traditional supplements or treatments often cannot match. Take, for example, collagen-boosting peptides. These are designed to stimulate the skin's production of collagen, a protein essential for elasticity and firmness. As we age, collagen breaks down, leading to sagging skin and wrinkles. By reintroducing peptides that trigger collagen production, the skin can regain some of its youthful resilience.

Then there are peptides like BPC-157, known for its powerful effects on healing and recovery. Athletes use it to support joint health and muscle recovery, while others benefit from its ability to reduce inflammation and speed up the body's natural healing processes. It's a multi-purpose peptide that showcases the body's potential when given the right tools to work with.

Additionally, peptides like Epitalon have shown potential in longevity studies, particularly for their effect on telomeres, the protective caps at the ends of chromosomes. As we age, these caps shorten, but studies suggest that Epitalon may help maintain telomere length, thereby supporting cellular health and potentially extending the lifespan of cells.

It's not just about looking younger—peptides offer a path to feeling younger, from the inside out. Imagine waking up energized, ready to take on the day with the kind of vigor you thought was lost to time. This is the promise of peptide-based anti-aging strategies, and it's why they're becoming an integral part of many people's routines.

How This Book Will Transform Your Routine

A journey into peptide therapy can feel overwhelming, especially with so much information available from different sources. This book is designed to be your trusted companion on that journey. Whether you're new to the world of anti-aging or looking to refine your approach, the content here will walk you through each step with clarity and practical guidance.

I'll begin with a comprehensive look at what peptides are, how they work, and why they are such a breakthrough in anti-aging. Following this foundational knowledge, i'll dive into the specifics of different peptide types, how they can be used safely, and the best protocols to maximize results. You'll learn about dosage, application methods, and the importance of stacking peptides to target multiple aspects of health simultaneously.

Beyond peptides, this book will also cover the complementary lifestyle changes that enhance their effects. From diet to exercise, sleep, and stress management, each of these factors plays a critical role in achieving the best possible results. You'll receive straightforward advice on integrating peptides into your daily life, along with insights into creating a balanced routine that supports long-term wellness.

Most importantly, this book provides a realistic approach. Peptides are not a magic bullet; they are part of a holistic strategy that requires consistency and care. We'll address the safety protocols, possible side effects, and the importance of choosing quality sources, so you can make informed decisions at every stage.

By the end, you'll not only have a full understanding of how peptides work but also a customized plan to incorporate them into your life. With practical tips, success stories, and scientifically backed information, this guide is here to empower you to take control of your health and embrace aging with confidence and grace. Let's begin this transformative journey together.

Chapter 1: Peptides and The Science of Aging

1.1 What Are Peptides and Why Are They Essential?

Imagine the body as a high-tech machine, filled with various parts that interact and communicate constantly to keep things running smoothly. This communication is crucial; every cell needs direction and purpose to function optimally. At the heart of this communication system are molecules like peptides, tiny but powerful agents that signal cells to carry out specific actions. To understand the role peptides play in our health, vitality, and aging process, let's dive into their structure, function, and their unique ability to impact how we age.

Peptides are often described as the building blocks of proteins, but they have a distinct identity and function. They are short chains of amino acids, typically consisting of between 2 and 50 amino acids, which makes them smaller and more flexible than proteins. This structure gives them an incredible versatility—they can travel through the body and attach to specific cells to send signals or trigger actions. This signaling function is what makes peptides so essential: they effectively communicate with cells to regulate physiological processes, from skin regeneration to hormone production, muscle repair, and immune response.

The Building Blocks of Life: Amino Acids and Peptides
To truly appreciate the role of peptides, we must first understand their components—amino acids. Amino acids are organic compounds that form the backbone of proteins and peptides, playing a vital role in virtually every biological process. There are 20 different amino acids in the human body, each with a unique structure and function. When amino acids link together in specific sequences, they create peptides. When these chains grow longer, they become proteins. Proteins are larger and more complex, carrying out heavy-duty tasks in the body. Peptides, however, are smaller and more specialized, acting as messengers to communicate specific instructions to cells.

Think of peptides as the "smart tech" within the body. While proteins may serve as the structure and machinery, peptides act like micro-managers, guiding, signaling, and supporting specific functions to keep the system balanced. Due to their smaller size, peptides can interact with cells more directly and effectively than larger molecules, allowing them to perform highly targeted roles.

The Essential Role of Peptides in the Human Body
Peptides are naturally occurring and essential for maintaining optimal health. They influence nearly every bodily system, from the nervous system to the immune system, skin, and

metabolism. Here's a breakdown of some of the critical functions peptides perform:

1. Skin Health and Repair

One of the most visible effects of peptides is on skin health. Certain peptides are responsible for signaling collagen production, a key protein that keeps skin firm, elastic, and youthful. As we age, collagen production declines, leading to wrinkles and sagging skin. Peptides help counteract this decline by stimulating collagen synthesis, effectively supporting skin regeneration and repair.

2. Hormone Regulation

Peptides play an essential role in the regulation of hormones, acting as precursors or stimulating the release of hormones that affect growth, metabolism, and reproductive functions. For example, Growth Hormone Releasing Peptide (GHRP) stimulates the production of human growth hormone (HGH), which is crucial for cell growth and regeneration.

3. Muscle Growth and Recovery

For athletes and fitness enthusiasts, peptides are significant due to their role in muscle growth, recovery, and performance. Certain peptides stimulate muscle protein synthesis, helping the body repair and grow muscle tissue after exercise. This process is vital not only for athletes but for anyone seeking to maintain muscle mass as they age.

4. Immune System Support

The immune system relies on peptides to fight infections and manage inflammation. Some peptides act as antimicrobial agents, directly combating bacteria, fungi, and viruses. Others support the immune response by reducing inflammation or signaling white blood cells to respond to an infection or injury.

5. Cognitive Function and Neuroprotection

Neuroprotective peptides have the unique ability to support brain health by protecting neurons from damage, reducing inflammation in the nervous system, and enhancing cognitive function. For individuals interested in preserving mental sharpness, these peptides can play a critical role in maintaining brain health as they age.

6. Metabolism and Weight Management

Peptides influence the body's metabolism by regulating fat breakdown, energy production, and appetite. Some peptides signal the release of hormones that help the body utilize fat for energy, making them a natural choice for those looking to manage their weight. They also play a role in blood sugar regulation, impacting insulin sensitivity and glucose uptake.

Peptides and the Aging Process

Aging, at its core, is a gradual decline in cellular function. Over time, cells lose their efficiency in repairing damage, producing energy, and communicating with one another. This decline manifests in the body through slower healing, decreased collagen production, reduced muscle mass, and less efficient immune responses. Peptides, by supporting and enhancing these processes, offer a promising approach to slowing or even reversing some of the signs of aging.

One of the main reasons peptides are effective in anti-aging is that they address issues at the cellular level. By signaling cells to regenerate, repair, or produce essential proteins, peptides can essentially "remind" the body to maintain its youthful functions. For instance, peptides that stimulate collagen production can help maintain the skin's elasticity and reduce the appearance of fine lines, while others that support muscle growth and repair can counteract the natural loss of muscle mass associated with aging.

This cellular-level impact is a fundamental reason peptides have gained popularity in anti-aging science. Unlike many products that merely mask aging on the surface, peptides work with the body's natural systems to support long-term vitality.

Why Peptides Are Essential in Modern Health and Wellness

In a world where health trends come and go, peptides stand out for their proven biological role and versatility. The more researchers uncover about peptides, the more applications emerge. Peptides aren't just a supplement or a skincare ingredient; they are an essential component of the body's signaling system. Here's why they have become a cornerstone in health and wellness today:

1. Highly Targeted and Specific

Peptides are designed to attach to specific receptors on cell surfaces, which means they can perform precise functions without widespread side effects. This specificity is rare in medicine and supplements, making peptides a valuable tool for targeted health support.

2. Synergistic with the Body's Natural Processes

Since peptides occur naturally in the body, they are generally well-tolerated and work synergistically with existing biological processes. Unlike synthetic compounds, peptides support the body's systems rather than override them, which can make them safer and more effective for long-term use.

3. Wide Range of Applications

From skincare to muscle growth, cognitive support to immune health, peptides offer solutions for a diverse array of health concerns. This adaptability makes them a powerful addition to a wellness routine, as they can be customized to fit specific needs.

4. Backed by Scientific Research

Peptides have been extensively studied in clinical and laboratory settings, with promising results for various health applications. Their safety and effectiveness are continually evaluated, contributing to an ever-growing body of knowledge that guides their use in health and wellness.

Different Types of Peptides and Their Unique Roles

As we delve deeper into the specifics of peptide types, it becomes clear that each peptide offers distinct benefits. Some of the most popular and well-researched peptides include:

Collagen-Boosting Peptides: Known for their role in skin health, these peptides stimulate the production of collagen and elastin, essential proteins that maintain skin elasticity and strength.

Growth Hormone Releasing Peptides (GHRPs): These peptides stimulate the release of growth hormone, supporting muscle growth, tissue repair, and overall cellular regeneration.

Thymosin Beta-4: Commonly used for its regenerative properties, this peptide plays a significant role in wound healing, tissue repair, and inflammation reduction.

BPC-157: Often called the "healing peptide," BPC-157 is known for its ability to support digestive health, muscle recovery, and overall tissue repair.

Epitalon: This peptide is studied for its effects on telomere length and longevity, as it may support cell lifespan and reduce age-related cellular decline.

The Role of Peptides in Enhancing Health and Youthfulness

Understanding peptides' foundational role in the body opens the door to a new way of approaching health and aging. They aren't merely supplements or enhancements; they're essential tools that help maintain the body's optimal function. Peptides represent a bridge between traditional wellness practices and cutting-edge science, allowing us to support our health in ways that align with natural processes.

1.2 Aging Demystified: How Peptides Counteract Cellular Decline

When we think of aging, we often focus on the physical signs—the gray hairs, the wrinkles, the stiffness in our joints. However, aging begins on a much smaller scale, deep within our cells, long before it becomes visible. Every process of aging, from the slow loss of muscle tone to the reduced elasticity of the skin, originates in cellular changes and declines in function. As cells age, they lose efficiency, resilience, and the ability to repair themselves, which collectively leads to the visible signs of aging we know well.

While aging is natural, our understanding of it has evolved, revealing insights into how we might delay or even counteract certain age-related changes. Peptides have emerged as a powerful ally in this pursuit, offering ways to support cellular health and resilience. To understand how peptides play a role in counteracting cellular decline, let's explore the science of aging itself, how cellular functions deteriorate over time, and the mechanisms through which peptides can support healthier aging.

The Cellular Basis of Aging

Cells are the building blocks of life, and their health directly influences how we age. Healthy cells are dynamic and capable of performing a wide range of functions—they produce energy, repair damage, and communicate with each other. However, as we age, these functions gradually weaken.

Several key factors contribute to cellular aging, including oxidative stress, DNA damage, telomere shortening, and reduced cellular communication. Over time, these factors accumulate and result in cellular dysfunction, which translates into the physical symptoms of aging.

1. Oxidative Stress and Free Radicals

Oxidative stress occurs when there is an imbalance between free radicals (unstable molecules that can damage cells) and antioxidants in the body. Free radicals are naturally produced during cellular processes like energy production, but they can also be increased by environmental factors like pollution and UV exposure. When left unchecked, these molecules can damage cell structures, proteins, and DNA, contributing to the signs of aging.

2. DNA Damage and Cellular Senescence

Our DNA is constantly under threat from various sources, including environmental toxins, UV radiation, and even normal cellular processes. When DNA becomes damaged, cells either repair the damage or, in cases of severe damage, become senescent. Senescent cells no longer function optimally and instead enter a "standby" mode where they cease dividing. While this is a protective mechanism to prevent damaged cells from proliferating, the buildup of senescent cells is a hallmark of aging and contributes to tissue degeneration.

3. Telomere Shortening

Telomeres are protective caps on the ends of chromosomes that prevent DNA from unraveling during cell division. Every time a cell divides, its telomeres become shorter. Eventually, when telomeres reach a critical length, the cell can no longer divide and becomes senescent. Telomere shortening is one of the clearest indicators of biological aging and is associated with age-related diseases.

4. Reduced Cellular Communication

As cells age, their ability to communicate with each other diminishes. Cellular communication is essential for coordinating various bodily functions, such as immune response and tissue repair. This decline in communication leads to a lack of synchrony among cells, resulting in less effective responses to damage and stress.

How Peptides Counteract Cellular Aging Mechanisms

Peptides have gained attention in the field of anti-aging because they directly support the body's natural ability to maintain cellular health and counteract the aging mechanisms described above. Unlike synthetic drugs, peptides are made up of naturally occurring amino acids that the body recognizes, allowing them to work in harmony with biological processes.

1. Antioxidant and Anti-Inflammatory Properties

Some peptides, like BPC-157, have been shown to reduce oxidative stress and inflammation, two significant contributors to cellular aging. By neutralizing free radicals and supporting the body's antioxidant defenses, these peptides help protect cells from the damage that accelerates aging. This can translate into healthier skin, reduced inflammation, and an overall decrease in age-related symptoms.

2. DNA Repair and Cellular Protection

Peptides like Epitalon have been studied for their potential to support DNA repair mechanisms. Epitalon, for instance, is believed to activate telomerase, an enzyme that helps maintain telomere length. By preserving telomere integrity, peptides may enable cells to continue dividing and functioning optimally for longer periods, effectively slowing down cellular aging.

3. Enhancing Cellular Communication

Certain peptides facilitate better cellular communication, ensuring that cells can coordinate and respond effectively to bodily needs. For example, peptides used in growth hormone stimulation, like GHRP (Growth Hormone Releasing Peptides), help improve cellular communication related to tissue growth and repair. Enhanced communication among cells supports more efficient healing and regeneration, two processes that typically decline with age.

4. Promoting Cellular Regeneration and Stem Cell Health

Peptides like Thymosin Beta-4 are known for their role in cellular regeneration and supporting stem cell function. Stem cells are unique cells with the ability to develop into various cell types and are vital for tissue repair. Peptides that promote stem cell health support the body's capacity to regenerate tissues, from muscle and skin to organs, which is crucial for maintaining vitality as we age.

Key Peptides in Counteracting Cellular Decline

Understanding the specific peptides involved in counteracting cellular aging can help us tailor peptide therapy to meet individual needs. Some of the key peptides known for their anti-aging properties are:

1. Epitalon

Epitalon is often referred to as a "longevity peptide" because of its role in telomere maintenance. Studies have shown that Epitalon can increase the activity of telomerase, the enzyme responsible for repairing and elongating telomeres. By supporting telomere health, Epitalon can effectively slow down cellular aging, contributing to improved cellular resilience and potentially extending lifespan.

2. BPC-157

Known as the "healing peptide," BPC-157 is renowned for its regenerative properties. It has been studied for its effects on muscle, joint, and gut health, where it aids in tissue repair and reduces inflammation. By minimizing inflammation and accelerating healing, BPC-157 helps reduce cellular stress, one of the primary contributors to aging.

3. Thymosin Beta-4

Thymosin Beta-4 is a peptide that plays a crucial role in wound healing and tissue regeneration. It promotes the migration of cells to injury sites, enhancing repair processes and supporting stem cell function. Its regenerative properties make it valuable in anti-aging, as it helps the body recover from injuries and maintain tissue health.

4. GHK-Cu (Copper Peptide)

Copper peptides, such as GHK-Cu, are celebrated for their skin-rejuvenating properties. GHK-Cu stimulates collagen synthesis and has been shown to improve skin elasticity and firmness. Additionally, GHK-Cu has antioxidant and anti-inflammatory properties, which help protect cells from oxidative damage, thus supporting a youthful appearance and cellular health.

5. CJC-1295 and Ipamorelin

These peptides are commonly used to increase growth hormone levels. Growth hormone plays a critical role in cellular regeneration, metabolism, and overall body composition. By stimulating growth hormone release, CJC-1295 and Ipamorelin support muscle growth, tissue repair, and metabolic health, all of which are vital for maintaining energy and vitality with age.

The Synergy Between Peptides and Cellular Health

While each peptide has specific functions, they can also work synergistically to provide comprehensive support for cellular health. Combining peptides that target various aspects of cellular aging, such as inflammation, telomere maintenance, and cellular communication, can produce more significant results. This approach, known as peptide stacking, is popular in anti-aging because it allows for a tailored protocol that addresses multiple factors of cellular decline simultaneously.

For example, a protocol that includes Epitalon for telomere health, BPC-157 for inflammation reduction, and Thymosin Beta-4 for tissue repair would provide broad-spectrum support to cells, addressing multiple aging pathways. This multi-faceted approach is what makes peptides such a valuable tool in anti-aging therapy—they can be customized to meet individual needs, offering support across the various cellular mechanisms that contribute to aging.

Embracing Peptide Therapy as a Holistic Approach to Aging

Counteracting cellular decline with peptides isn't about reversing the clock entirely but about promoting resilience, health, and vitality. Peptides support the body in maintaining its natural repair and regenerative processes, helping us age with strength and energy. They provide a bridge between traditional health practices and modern science, allowing us to work with our biology rather than against it.

Embracing peptide therapy as part of a holistic approach to aging means looking beyond quick fixes and understanding that sustainable results come from supporting cellular health over time. By combining peptide therapy with healthy lifestyle choices—such as a balanced diet, regular exercise, quality sleep, and stress management—we can create a solid foundation for longevity.

1.3 Decoding the Link Between Peptides and Longevity

When we talk about longevity, we're not just talking about adding years to life but about enhancing those years with health, vitality, and resilience. The dream of living longer without sacrificing quality of life is one that scientists and wellness enthusiasts alike have pursued for centuries. While genetics play a significant role in lifespan, modern research shows that our environment, lifestyle, and even our internal biological processes can be influenced to improve both the length and quality of our lives. Among the promising tools for this purpose, peptides have gained considerable attention for their potential to support longevity.

Peptides work on a cellular level, which means they have the potential to influence processes tied directly to aging and health span (the period of life spent in good health). They do this by engaging in activities that enhance cell repair, reduce oxidative stress, maintain metabolic function, and even support the immune system. In this section, we will decode the link between peptides and longevity, exploring how peptides can support healthier, longer lives by impacting crucial biological pathways.

Understanding Longevity at the Cellular Level

Longevity begins at the cellular level. Our cells are responsible for every function in the body, from energy production and immune defense to tissue repair and brain function. As we age, our cells encounter various challenges that reduce their efficiency and resilience. Here are some primary processes that contribute to aging and how peptides can help address them:

1. Cellular Senescence

Cellular senescence is a state in which cells lose the ability to divide and function optimally. Senescent cells are sometimes called "zombie cells" because, although they're still alive, they no longer contribute to the body's functionality. These cells can release inflammatory signals that affect surrounding healthy cells, accelerating the aging process. Peptides like Epitalon have shown promise in reducing cellular senescence by promoting telomerase activity, which helps maintain telomere length and cellular health.

2. Oxidative Stress and Free Radical Damage

Oxidative stress occurs when free radicals, which are unstable molecules produced through normal cellular processes, accumulate and cause damage to cell structures, DNA, and proteins. Peptides with antioxidant properties, such as GHK-Cu, help neutralize free radicals, protecting cells from oxidative damage that accelerates aging.

3. Decline in Mitochondrial Function

Mitochondria are the powerhouses of cells, producing the energy necessary for cellular function. As we age, mitochondrial function tends to decline, which leads to reduced energy levels and an accumulation of damage within the cells. Peptides that stimulate mitochondrial health or energy production can support longevity by helping cells maintain optimal energy levels.

4. Telomere Shortening

Telomeres are the protective caps at the ends of chromosomes that prevent DNA from unraveling during cell division. Each time a cell divides, the telomeres shorten, eventually reaching a point where the cell can no longer divide and becomes senescent. Peptides like Epitalon are studied for their potential role in activating telomerase, an enzyme that replenishes telomere length, thus supporting cell viability over a more extended period.

By addressing these core aspects of cellular health, peptides provide the body with tools to maintain youthfulness and vitality. This cellular approach is why peptides are uniquely suited for supporting longevity.

How Peptides Influence Key Longevity Pathways

To understand how peptides influence longevity, it's helpful to look at some of the main biological pathways that impact aging and lifespan. Scientists have identified several pathways that regulate how the body ages, and peptides have shown potential in modulating these pathways.

1. AMPK Pathway (Energy and Metabolism)

AMPK (adenosine monophosphate-activated protein kinase) is an enzyme that plays a role in cellular energy balance. It helps cells take in and use glucose and fatty acids for energy, which is essential for metabolism and energy production. Certain peptides support AMPK activity, promoting energy efficiency at the cellular level. This not only supports physical vitality but also enhances metabolic health, which is crucial for longevity.

2. mTOR Pathway (Growth and Regeneration)

The mTOR (mechanistic target of rapamycin) pathway is involved in cell growth, proliferation, and protein synthesis. While the mTOR pathway is essential for growth, overactivity has been linked to accelerated aging and age-related diseases. Some peptides, particularly those related to growth hormone stimulation, can influence the mTOR pathway, supporting regeneration without overstimulation. By managing mTOR activity, these peptides help balance cellular growth with longevity.

3. SIRT1 Pathway (DNA Repair and Protection)

SIRT1 is a protein associated with DNA repair, cellular stress response, and mitochondrial function. It is part of a group of proteins known as sirtuins, which have been linked to longevity. Peptides that support SIRT1 activity help enhance DNA repair mechanisms, protect cells from stress, and maintain mitochondrial health. This pathway is crucial for supporting longevity on a genetic and cellular level.

4. Telomerase Activation (Chromosome Stability)

Telomerase is the enzyme responsible for replenishing telomeres, the protective caps on chromosomes. Epitalon, for example, has been studied for its role in activating telomerase, which supports telomere length and, consequently, cell lifespan. By maintaining telomere integrity, telomerase activation helps prevent cellular senescence, one of the most significant contributors to aging.

The Future of Peptide Therapy and Longevity Research

The use of peptides to support longevity is an evolving field, with new studies continually emerging to expand our understanding. Researchers are exploring how peptides can be used alongside other anti-aging interventions, such as gene therapy and stem cell research, to further enhance health span and life span.

One promising area of research is the potential for peptides to support "biological reprogramming," a process that aims to reset cells to a more youthful state without the risks of gene manipulation. The idea is that, by providing cells with the right signals—such as those delivered by peptides—they can return to a more youthful functioning level, reducing the accumulation of age-related damage.

As the field advances, peptides may become more refined and targeted, allowing for highly personalized peptide therapies that address specific genetic markers or health concerns. This level of precision could revolutionize how we approach aging, offering people a tailored path to longevity.

Embracing a Peptide-Based Longevity Routine

For those interested in pursuing longevity, the idea of a peptide-based routine offers an accessible, natural approach.

Unlike many invasive anti-aging treatments, peptides work with the body's systems, supporting natural processes rather than disrupting them. The benefits of peptides for longevity are cumulative, meaning that consistency and commitment over time are essential.

When integrating peptides into a longevity routine, it's essential to consult with a healthcare provider experienced in peptide therapy. They can help you choose peptides tailored to your health goals, determine appropriate dosages, and monitor your progress. Additionally, combining peptides with lifestyle practices, such as a nutritious diet, regular exercise, stress management, and quality sleep, maximizes their impact.

Chapter 2: Exploring the Anti-Aging Peptide Family

2.1 GHK-Cu – The Skin Rejuvenator

Imagine waking up, looking in the mirror, and noticing smoother, firmer, and more radiant skin—a complexion that reflects the energy and youthfulness you feel inside. For many, achieving that vibrant, youthful appearance without invasive procedures or complicated regimens is a top skincare goal. This is where GHK-Cu, often referred to as "the skin rejuvenator peptide," becomes relevant. Known for its remarkable ability to enhance skin elasticity, firmness, and overall health, GHK-Cu has earned its place as one of the most popular peptides in the anti-aging industry.

But what makes GHK-Cu so effective? This powerful tripeptide, made up of the amino acids glycine, histidine, and lysine, combined with a copper ion, functions as a signaler in the skin, instructing cells to repair damage, produce collagen,

and combat oxidative stress. These actions directly address many common signs of aging, such as wrinkles, fine lines, and loss of elasticity, making GHK-Cu a compelling choice for anyone looking to maintain youthful skin.
Whether you're new to peptides or a seasoned skincare enthusiast, understanding GHK-Cu's mechanism of action can provide valuable insight into how it supports healthy, resilient skin.

What is GHK-Cu?

GHK-Cu is a naturally occurring peptide found in human plasma, saliva, and urine, and its levels decrease with age. In its natural form, GHK-Cu is primarily involved in wound healing, immune response, and tissue repair. What makes GHK-Cu unique is its affinity for copper, a mineral that plays an essential role in cellular repair and regeneration.

The "Cu" in GHK-Cu stands for copper, which binds to the peptide, giving it a distinctive blue color when in solution. Copper is a vital trace element that, when paired with GHK, forms a complex capable of delivering powerful anti-aging benefits. This combination is effective because copper supports collagen synthesis, promotes wound healing, and acts as an antioxidant, while GHK enhances copper's ability to penetrate the skin and deliver these benefits directly to cells.

As a tripeptide, GHK-Cu is small enough to penetrate the skin effectively, making it ideal for topical applications. When applied to the skin, GHK-Cu binds to receptors on skin cells, sending signals to initiate repair processes. This is why it's commonly found in anti-aging skincare products, where it's used to support collagen production, increase skin elasticity, and reduce visible signs of aging.

How GHK-Cu Works: The Science of Skin Rejuvenation

To appreciate the impact of GHK-Cu on skin health, it's helpful to understand how skin aging occurs on a cellular level. As we age, our skin's ability to repair itself diminishes. Collagen production slows down, elastin (the protein responsible for skin's "snap-back" quality) begins to break down, and the skin's natural antioxidant defenses weaken. This leads to the formation of wrinkles, fine lines, and sagging skin.

GHK-Cu counters these effects by initiating several biological processes that directly impact skin structure and resilience:

1. Stimulating Collagen and Glycosaminoglycan Synthesis
Collagen is a primary structural protein in the skin, providing firmness and support. Glycosaminoglycans (such as hyaluronic acid) help retain moisture, keeping skin plump and hydrated. GHK-Cu has been shown to increase collagen synthesis, which improves skin's structural integrity, reduces wrinkles, and enhances overall firmness. Additionally, by promoting glycosaminoglycan production, GHK-Cu helps improve hydration and smoothness, giving skin a youthful, healthy glow.

2. Promoting Skin Cell Regeneration and Wound Healing

One of GHK-Cu's original medical uses was in wound healing due to its ability to encourage cell regeneration. It accelerates the repair of damaged skin by promoting the proliferation of fibroblasts, which are cells responsible for producing collagen and elastin. This regenerative effect is beneficial for anti-aging because it supports continuous cell turnover, maintaining fresh, healthy skin.

3. Reducing Inflammation and Oxidative Stress

Inflammation and oxidative stress are two major contributors to skin aging. GHK-Cu has demonstrated anti-inflammatory properties, helping reduce redness, irritation, and other signs of inflammation that can accelerate aging. Furthermore, GHK-Cu acts as an antioxidant, neutralizing free radicals that cause oxidative damage. This dual action protects skin cells from environmental stressors like UV exposure and pollution, which can lead to premature aging.

4. Enhancing Skin Barrier Function

The skin barrier is essential for retaining moisture and protecting against external pollutants. GHK-Cu supports the skin's barrier function by encouraging lipid synthesis, which strengthens the outermost layer of skin. A healthy skin barrier not only improves hydration but also enhances the skin's resilience to environmental stressors, helping it stay supple and smooth.

Benefits of GHK-Cu for Aging Skin

The advantages of GHK-Cu extend beyond mere aesthetics; they go to the heart of what defines healthy, youthful skin. By addressing aging on multiple fronts, GHK-Cu offers a comprehensive approach to skin rejuvenation. Here are some of the key benefits that make GHK-Cu a go-to peptide for anti-aging:

1. Smoother, Firmer Skin
With its ability to stimulate collagen production and reduce inflammation, GHK-Cu helps smooth fine lines and wrinkles, giving the skin a firmer, more lifted appearance. Regular use of GHK-Cu in skincare products has been shown to significantly improve skin texture, making it smoother to the touch.

2. Enhanced Skin Elasticity
Elasticity is what allows skin to "snap back" after being stretched. GHK-Cu supports the production of elastin, a protein that provides this quality. By improving elastin levels, GHK-Cu helps maintain skin's youthful bounce and resilience, reducing the appearance of sagging and wrinkles.

3. Increased Hydration and Plumpness
By promoting glycosaminoglycan synthesis, GHK-Cu enhances skin's ability to retain moisture. This increase in hydration keeps skin looking plump and reduces the visibility of fine lines, as hydrated skin appears fuller and healthier.

4. Protection Against Environmental Damage

GHK-Cu's antioxidant properties help protect skin from environmental stressors that contribute to aging. By neutralizing free radicals, GHK-Cu reduces oxidative stress, shielding skin cells from damage caused by factors like UV radiation, pollution, and toxins.

5. Accelerated Healing and Reduced Scarring

Because of its regenerative properties, GHK-Cu is beneficial for reducing scars, spots, and blemishes. It promotes faster healing and can improve the appearance of acne scars, hyperpigmentation, and other imperfections, leaving skin with a more even tone and texture.

How to Use GHK-Cu in Your Skincare Routine

Incorporating GHK-Cu into your skincare routine can be as simple as selecting products that contain this peptide, such as serums, creams, or face masks. Here are some tips for getting the most out of GHK-Cu in your skincare routine:

1. Start with Clean Skin

For GHK-Cu to penetrate effectively, it's best applied to clean skin. Start your routine with a gentle cleanser to remove any dirt, oil, or makeup. Pat your face dry before applying products that contain GHK-Cu.

2. Layer with Other Hydrating Ingredients

GHK-Cu works well with hydrating ingredients like hyaluronic acid, which can enhance the peptide's effects.

After applying GHK-Cu, follow with a moisturizer to lock in hydration and strengthen the skin barrier.

3. Use Consistently
Consistency is key when it comes to skincare. For visible results, apply GHK-Cu products regularly, typically once or twice a day as recommended by the product instructions. It may take a few weeks to notice significant changes, but patience will yield results.

4. Combine with Sunscreen
To maximize the anti-aging effects of GHK-Cu, always use sunscreen during the day. Sun protection is crucial for preventing further damage, as UV rays can accelerate collagen breakdown and oxidative stress. Applying GHK-Cu at night and following with sunscreen in the morning creates a powerful anti-aging routine.

Safety and Potential Side Effects of GHK-Cu

While GHK-Cu is generally considered safe, especially when used topically, it's always wise to conduct a patch test to ensure there's no adverse reaction. Some individuals may experience mild irritation or redness, particularly if they have sensitive skin. To test for sensitivity, apply a small amount of the product to an inconspicuous area, such as the inner arm, and wait 24 hours to see if any reaction occurs.

As with any skincare ingredient, moderation is important. Overuse of products containing GHK-Cu can lead to overstimulation, which may cause redness or irritation. It's best to follow product instructions carefully and consult a dermatologist if you have any concerns, especially if you're prone to skin conditions or have allergies.

The Future of GHK-Cu in Anti-Aging Skincare

As science continues to explore the mechanisms of aging, GHK-Cu is likely to remain at the forefront of anti-aging skincare due to its multi-functional benefits. With a growing body of research supporting its efficacy in collagen production, antioxidant activity, and wound healing, GHK-Cu may even find expanded applications in regenerative medicine beyond skincare.

In the years ahead, we may see more advanced formulations of GHK-Cu, combined with other bioactive compounds, to create powerful anti-aging treatments. These developments could unlock even more potential for GHK-Cu, making it an essential component not only for those focused on anti-aging but also for individuals interested in maintaining overall skin health.

2.2 BPC-157 – The Healing Accelerator

The search for effective and safe healing solutions has been an age-old quest, with countless people seeking ways to alleviate pain, repair injuries, and enhance physical resilience. In recent years, BPC-157, often called "the healing accelerator," has gained significant attention for its unique and potent regenerative properties. Originally derived from a protein found in the stomach, BPC-157 has a natural affinity for healing and is celebrated for its ability to support tissue repair, reduce inflammation, and promote recovery in ways that few other peptides can match.

BPC-157 is short for "Body Protection Compound 157," and its name highlights its primary function—protecting and healing the body. This peptide has been studied for its impressive effects on various tissues, including muscles, tendons, ligaments, and even organs like the stomach and intestines. With applications that range from accelerating recovery after workouts to promoting wound healing and supporting joint health, BPC-157 stands out as a versatile tool for anyone interested in both anti-aging and physical wellness.

What is BPC-157?

BPC-157 is a pentadecapeptide, meaning it is composed of 15 amino acids. This relatively simple structure allows it to interact with a wide range of cells and tissues, promoting healing in various areas of the body. While it was initially identified in the stomach, where it plays a role in protecting and repairing the stomach lining, research has shown that BPC-157's benefits extend far beyond gastrointestinal health. It has been found to support everything from muscle recovery to tendon and ligament repair, making it an attractive option for athletes, active individuals, and anyone dealing with chronic injuries.

What makes BPC-157 unique is that it is both naturally occurring and highly specific in its actions. Unlike some synthetic compounds, BPC-157 works harmoniously with the body's natural processes, enhancing healing without interfering with other bodily functions. Its safety profile, combined with its effectiveness, has made it a popular choice in the field of regenerative medicine.

How BPC-157 Works: The Science of Regeneration and Recovery

At its core, BPC-157 operates by interacting with various growth factors and receptors within the body, essentially "instructing" cells to repair and regenerate. This peptide accelerates the healing process through several mechanisms:

1. Enhancing Blood Vessel Formation (Angiogenesis)

BPC-157 is known for its ability to promote angiogenesis, the formation of new blood vessels. Blood vessels are crucial for delivering oxygen, nutrients, and immune cells to damaged tissues, which supports faster healing. By stimulating angiogenesis, BPC-157 ensures that injured areas receive an adequate supply of resources necessary for recovery.

2. Reducing Inflammation

Inflammation is a natural part of the healing process, but excessive or chronic inflammation can delay recovery and lead to tissue damage. BPC-157 has been shown to reduce inflammation in various tissues, helping to minimize pain, swelling, and redness. This anti-inflammatory effect allows for faster healing by preventing prolonged immune responses that can otherwise damage healthy tissues.

3. Stimulating Growth Factors and Collagen Production

BPC-157 promotes the activity of growth factors, which are proteins that play a crucial role in cellular repair and regeneration. Growth factors, such as VEGF (vascular endothelial growth factor) and FGF (fibroblast growth factor), are essential for tissue healing, and BPC-157 helps enhance their production. Additionally, BPC-157 encourages collagen synthesis, which is vital for maintaining the structural integrity of skin, tendons, ligaments, and other connective tissues.

4. Supporting Cellular Communication and Tissue Repair

Another remarkable aspect of BPC-157 is its ability to enhance cellular communication, allowing cells to coordinate more effectively during the healing process. This ensures that damaged tissues receive the necessary cellular support for efficient repair and regeneration. BPC-157 also encourages the migration of fibroblasts, which are cells involved in the formation of connective tissue, to injury sites.

5. Protecting Gastrointestinal Health

BPC-157's origin in the stomach means it is particularly effective at supporting gastrointestinal health. It has been shown to promote healing of the stomach lining, reduce symptoms of inflammatory bowel disease, and even repair damage caused by ulcers. This makes BPC-157 especially useful for individuals dealing with digestive issues, as it can support both the stomach and intestinal health.

Benefits of BPC-157 for Healing and Recovery

Given its wide-ranging effects on different types of tissues, BPC-157 offers numerous benefits for those interested in anti-aging, recovery, and overall wellness. Here's a closer look at how BPC-157 can support various aspects of health:

1. Enhanced Muscle Recovery

BPC-157 is particularly popular among athletes and fitness enthusiasts due to its ability to accelerate muscle recovery. After intense workouts, muscles experience microtears that require time and resources to repair. By improving blood flow, reducing inflammation, and promoting cellular repair, BPC-157 helps muscles recover more quickly, allowing for better performance and reduced downtime.

2. Joint and Ligament Health

Aging and physical activity can take a toll on joints, tendons, and ligaments, often leading to discomfort or injury. BPC-157 supports the health of these tissues by stimulating collagen synthesis and reducing inflammation. Regular use of BPC-157 has been associated with improved joint mobility, reduced pain, and better resilience against strain or injury.

3. Accelerated Wound Healing

BPC-157 has been shown to promote faster wound healing, making it beneficial for anyone dealing with cuts, abrasions, or post-surgical recovery. By encouraging cell migration and collagen production, BPC-157 helps wounds close more quickly and minimizes scarring, supporting skin regeneration and health.

4. Improved Digestive Health

Due to its origins in the stomach, BPC-157 is highly effective at supporting digestive health. It has been studied for its ability to heal ulcers, reduce symptoms of inflammatory bowel disease, and repair damage to the stomach lining. This makes BPC-157 an appealing option for individuals with chronic digestive issues or those seeking to improve their gut health.

5. Reduction of Chronic Inflammation

Chronic inflammation is a common issue that contributes to various health problems, including joint pain, digestive issues, and skin conditions. BPC-157's anti-inflammatory properties help mitigate chronic inflammation, supporting long-term health and reducing the risk of inflammation-related aging signs.

6. Protection Against Organ Damage

Interestingly, BPC-157 has also shown promise in protecting organs like the liver and kidneys from damage caused by toxins or injury. Studies have indicated that BPC-157 can reduce oxidative stress and inflammation in these organs, suggesting that it may be helpful for individuals looking to protect their internal health as they age.

Integrating BPC-157 Into Your Wellness Routine

Using BPC-157 effectively requires an understanding of its application methods, dosages, and safety protocols. While

BPC-157 is most commonly available as an injectable peptide, topical and oral forms are also becoming more accessible.

1. Injectable BPC-157

The most popular and effective method for using BPC-157 is through subcutaneous or intramuscular injections, which deliver the peptide directly into the bloodstream. Injections are generally administered close to the area of injury or discomfort for targeted effects, though systemic benefits can also be achieved through regular injections. Consulting with a healthcare provider can ensure proper technique and dosage.

2. Topical BPC-157

For those interested in skin or surface-level healing, BPC-157 creams or gels can be applied topically to areas that need repair, such as wounds, scars, or inflammation sites. While topical applications may not penetrate as deeply as injections, they still provide localized benefits.

3. Oral BPC-157

BPC-157 is also available in oral forms, which are primarily used for gastrointestinal health. Taken orally, BPC-157 can target the stomach and intestines more effectively, supporting healing from within the digestive tract. This method is ideal for individuals dealing with ulcers or inflammatory bowel conditions.

Potential Side Effects and Safety Considerations

BPC-157 is generally well-tolerated, especially when used within recommended doses. However, as with any supplement or therapy, there are potential side effects to consider. Some users report mild discomfort at the injection site or, occasionally, symptoms like nausea or dizziness. These reactions are typically mild and short-lived.

To minimize the risk of side effects, it's advisable to consult a healthcare provider experienced in peptide therapy, particularly if you have any pre-existing medical conditions. BPC-157's safety profile is strong, but as with all treatments, it's best used under professional supervision to ensure optimal results and safety.

The Future of BPC-157 in Regenerative Medicine

Research into BPC-157 continues to expand, with new studies exploring its potential applications in fields beyond traditional healing. Scientists are investigating BPC-157's effects on brain health, liver protection, and even nerve regeneration, which could open doors to innovative treatments for neurodegenerative diseases and other chronic conditions.

With its ability to promote natural healing processes and reduce inflammation, BPC-157 may become an integral part of holistic health practices. It represents a future where medicine not only treats symptoms but also supports the body's innate ability to repair itself. As science progresses, BPC-157's role in both preventive and regenerative medicine may broaden, making it a cornerstone for those seeking longevity, resilience, and sustained health.

2.3 Epitalon – The Longevity Enhancer

Imagine a life where the effects of aging are slowed, vitality is preserved, and the cells of the body remain resilient for years beyond what we've come to expect. In the field of longevity science, Epitalon has become an area of intense interest due to its potential to promote these exact outcomes. Often referred to as "the longevity enhancer," Epitalon stands out as a peptide known for its unique impact on the aging process, specifically through its role in telomerase activation—a function that may support cellular longevity and, consequently, extend lifespan.

Epitalon, a synthetic tetrapeptide, was developed based on the work of Russian scientist Vladimir Khavinson, who studied its effects on aging. It is derived from Epithalamin, a naturally occurring peptide in the pineal gland, which has been linked to regulating aging processes and cellular health. Research into Epitalon has shown that it can stimulate telomerase production, an enzyme responsible for maintaining telomeres, the protective caps on chromosomes. Because telomeres shorten with each cell division, they are closely associated with cellular aging. By supporting telomere length, Epitalon may offer a path to healthier, more resilient cells and, potentially, a longer life.

What is Epitalon?

Epitalon (also known as Epithalon) is a tetrapeptide, meaning it consists of four amino acids: alanine, glutamic acid, aspartic acid, and glycine. This simple structure belies its profound impact on cellular health, particularly through its influence on telomerase, the enzyme that rebuilds and maintains telomeres. Telomeres are the protective "caps" at the ends of chromosomes, and their length serves as a marker for cellular aging. Each time a cell divides, its telomeres shorten until they reach a critical length, at which point the cell can no longer divide and becomes senescent or dies. This process is a major contributor to aging and age-related diseases.

Epitalon's unique ability to activate telomerase production helps slow down this shortening of telomeres, which may allow cells to continue dividing and functioning optimally for a longer period. By protecting telomere length, Epitalon could, theoretically, delay the onset of cellular aging, contributing to an extended health span—the period of life spent in good health. This potential to preserve cellular vitality has earned Epitalon its reputation as a "longevity enhancer," and it has been the focus of various studies exploring its effects on aging, immunity, and overall well-being.

How Epitalon Works: The Science of Telomeres and Telomerase

To understand how Epitalon contributes to longevity, it's essential to examine the function of telomeres and the role telomerase plays in maintaining these structures. Telomeres are like the protective plastic tips at the end of shoelaces; they prevent chromosomes from deteriorating or sticking to each other, which can lead to cellular malfunction or death. However, each time a cell divides, a small portion of the telomere is lost, causing them to shorten over time.

Telomerase, an enzyme naturally produced by certain cells, can rebuild telomeres, effectively countering the shortening process. Unfortunately, telomerase production is typically low in most cells and decreases further with age. Epitalon works by stimulating the production of telomerase, which can restore telomere length and potentially rejuvenate cells. This telomere-preserving action is crucial for longevity because it allows cells to continue dividing and functioning without entering senescence, the "standby" state associated with aging and cellular decline.

Beyond telomerase activation, Epitalon also influences several other biological processes that support longevity:

1. Regulation of Circadian Rhythms

Epitalon is derived from the pineal gland, an organ responsible for regulating melatonin production, which in turn affects circadian rhythms. Studies have shown that Epitalon can help normalize melatonin levels and improve sleep patterns, particularly in older adults. By supporting healthy sleep-wake cycles, Epitalon contributes to better overall health and recovery, both of which are essential for longevity.

2. Antioxidant Activity

Epitalon has demonstrated antioxidant properties, helping neutralize free radicals that cause oxidative stress. Oxidative stress damages cells and accelerates aging, so reducing this stress is critical for maintaining cellular health. By combating oxidative damage, Epitalon supports the body's natural defenses against aging.

3. Immune System Support

Aging is often associated with a decline in immune function, which increases susceptibility to infections and diseases. Epitalon has been shown to enhance immune function, making it a valuable tool for those seeking to maintain a robust immune system as they age.

Benefits of Epitalon for Longevity and Anti-Aging

Epitalon's ability to support telomere length and enhance cellular health offers a range of benefits for those interested in aging more gracefully and maintaining vitality. Here's how Epitalon contributes to various aspects of health:

1. Delayed Cellular Aging

By promoting telomerase activity, Epitalon helps protect telomere length, which is directly linked to cellular lifespan. Longer telomeres allow cells to continue dividing, supporting tissue health and reducing the likelihood of age-related cellular decline. This preservation of cellular function is one of the primary reasons Epitalon is considered a longevity peptide.

2. Improved Sleep and Circadian Rhythms

Epitalon's influence on melatonin production and the regulation of circadian rhythms can lead to better sleep quality. As we age, sleep patterns often become disrupted, leading to poor recovery and increased stress on the body. By supporting a natural sleep cycle, Epitalon enhances recovery and reduces the wear and tear associated with poor sleep.

3. Enhanced Immune Function

With aging, the immune system tends to weaken, increasing vulnerability to infections and chronic illnesses. Epitalon has been shown to strengthen immune function, helping the body resist infections and recover more efficiently. This immune support is critical for healthy aging and longevity.

4. Reduced Oxidative Stress

Epitalon's antioxidant effects help protect cells from oxidative damage, a major contributor to aging. By neutralizing free radicals, Epitalon reduces cellular stress and supports DNA stability, further preserving cell health and vitality.

5. Potential for Disease Prevention

Because Epitalon helps preserve cellular function and immune health, it may play a role in preventing age-related diseases. While research is ongoing, Epitalon's support for cellular resilience could reduce the risk of diseases like cardiovascular disease, neurodegeneration, and metabolic disorders, all of which are closely linked to aging.

Integrating Epitalon into a Longevity Routine

Epitalon is commonly administered through subcutaneous injections, allowing the peptide to enter the bloodstream directly and exert its effects efficiently. When incorporating Epitalon into a longevity regimen, it's essential to consult a healthcare provider experienced in peptide therapy to determine the appropriate dosage and frequency.

1. Dosage and Administration

Epitalon is typically administered in cycles, with users receiving injections over a period (often two to four weeks) followed by a break. The dosage and frequency can vary depending on individual health goals and needs, so professional guidance is advised. Following recommended protocols ensures safe and effective use.

2. Supporting Lifestyle Practices

To maximize the effects of Epitalon, it's beneficial to pair it with a healthy lifestyle. Regular exercise, a balanced diet rich in antioxidants, quality sleep, and stress management are all important for promoting longevity. Epitalon can amplify the benefits of these practices, creating a holistic approach to anti-aging.

3. Monitoring and Adjusting

As with any peptide therapy, it's advisable to monitor results and adjust the regimen as needed. Blood tests, health check-ups, and consultations with a healthcare provider can help track the impact of Epitalon on health markers and ensure optimal outcomes.

Potential Side Effects and Safety Considerations

Epitalon has been extensively studied and is generally well-tolerated when used within recommended dosages. However, as with any supplement or therapy, it's essential to be aware of potential side effects. Some individuals may experience mild reactions, such as temporary fatigue or digestive discomfort. These side effects are usually minor and short-lived.

To minimize the risk of side effects, it's best to follow a healthcare provider's instructions and avoid exceeding recommended dosages. Epitalon's safety profile is strong, especially compared to many pharmaceutical anti-aging treatments, making it an appealing choice for those seeking a natural approach to longevity.

The Future of Epitalon in Anti-Aging Research

The study of Epitalon continues to advance, with researchers exploring its potential applications in new areas of health and longevity. Some scientists are investigating whether Epitalon can be used in combination with other peptides to amplify its effects, while others are studying its impact on specific age-related diseases. As our understanding of telomeres, telomerase, and aging progresses, Epitalon may play an even greater role in anti-aging therapies.

With the promise of maintaining cellular health and resilience, Epitalon represents an exciting frontier in the quest for longevity. It reflects a shift in anti-aging science—from focusing solely on symptom management to supporting the body's natural mechanisms for health and vitality.

2.4 Thymosin Beta-4 – Immunity and Recovery

In the journey of healthy aging, two of the most important factors to maintain are a robust immune system and a body that can recover swiftly from physical stress, injury, or illness. This is where Thymosin Beta-4 (TB4), a peptide celebrated for its role in immunity and recovery, takes center stage. Known for its regenerative properties, Thymosin Beta-4 aids in wound healing, inflammation reduction, and immune support, making it a powerful ally for those seeking to age gracefully and maintain vitality.

Thymosin Beta-4 is a naturally occurring peptide produced by the thymus gland, an organ that plays a crucial role in immune function. As we age, our immune response gradually weakens, leading to increased vulnerability to infections, slower recovery times, and a greater likelihood of chronic inflammation. Thymosin Beta-4 has been shown to address these concerns by supporting immune cell activity, promoting tissue repair, and reducing inflammation—processes that are essential for staying active and resilient as we age..

What is Thymosin Beta-4?

Thymosin Beta-4 is a peptide made up of 43 amino acids. It is naturally present in most tissues and is particularly abundant in areas that require rapid cell turnover, such as the skin, eyes, heart, and muscles. TB4 was initially discovered in the thymus gland, where it plays a role in immune system regulation, but research has since revealed its broader regenerative capabilities. Thymosin Beta-4 is released by cells in response to injury, where it acts as a signaling molecule to promote healing and reduce inflammation.

What sets Thymosin Beta-4 apart from other peptides is its ability to travel throughout the body, reaching damaged tissues and helping to coordinate repair processes. Unlike peptides that target specific areas, Thymosin Beta-4 operates on a systemic level, making it versatile for both injury recovery and general immune support. Its ability to interact with a wide range of cell types allows it to promote healing in various tissues, from skin and muscles to organs and connective tissues.

How Thymosin Beta-4 Works: The Science of Immunity and Tissue Repair

Thymosin Beta-4's influence on immunity and recovery is rooted in its interaction with several biological processes, including cellular migration, inflammation modulation, and tissue regeneration. When injury or infection occurs, TB4 is released to help repair the affected area and minimize inflammation, ensuring that the body can recover effectively without prolonged immune activation.

Here are the key mechanisms by which Thymosin Beta-4 promotes immunity and tissue repair:

1. Promoting Cellular Migration

One of Thymosin Beta-4's primary functions is to encourage the migration of cells to sites of injury or inflammation. TB4 stimulates the movement of fibroblasts (cells that produce collagen and extracellular matrix) and endothelial cells (which line blood vessels), both of which are crucial for wound healing. This cellular migration ensures that damaged tissues receive the necessary resources to repair and regenerate, which is especially valuable in maintaining skin elasticity, muscle tone, and overall tissue integrity.

2. Reducing Inflammation and Oxidative Stress

Inflammation is a natural part of the body's response to injury or infection, but excessive or chronic inflammation can lead to tissue damage and slow recovery. Thymosin Beta-4 has demonstrated anti-inflammatory effects, helping to regulate immune responses and reduce oxidative stress. By moderating inflammation, TB4 allows the body to heal without the risk of prolonged immune activation, which can otherwise lead to chronic pain, swelling, and other issues associated with aging.

3. Stimulating Angiogenesis (Blood Vessel Formation)

Blood flow is essential for healing, as it delivers oxygen, nutrients, and immune cells to damaged tissues. Thymosin Beta-4 promotes angiogenesis, the formation of new blood vessels, which ensures that injured areas receive an adequate blood supply for faster healing. This increase in blood flow also supports better skin health and vitality, as well as improved muscle recovery after exercise or injury.

4. Encouraging Stem Cell Differentiation and Tissue Regeneration

Stem cells are unique cells with the potential to develop into different cell types, which is essential for tissue repair and regeneration. Thymosin Beta-4 supports stem cell differentiation, enabling the body to replace damaged cells more efficiently. This regenerative effect is beneficial for maintaining youthful skin, strong muscles, and resilient organs, all of which contribute to a higher quality of life as we age.

5. Supporting Immune Cell Activity

Thymosin Beta-4 plays an essential role in regulating the activity of immune cells, including T-cells, which are crucial for defending against infections and maintaining immune balance. TB4 enhances immune function, helping the body respond to pathogens while avoiding overactive immune responses that can lead to chronic inflammation. This immune support is particularly valuable for older adults, whose immune systems often become less responsive with age.

Benefits of Thymosin Beta-4 for Immunity and Recovery

Thymosin Beta-4's broad range of effects makes it a valuable tool for enhancing immunity, promoting recovery, and supporting overall wellness. Here's how TB4 can contribute to various aspects of health:

1. Accelerated Wound Healing

Thymosin Beta-4's ability to promote cellular migration and blood vessel formation allows for faster wound healing. Whether it's a cut, abrasion, or post-surgical recovery, TB4 helps tissues repair efficiently, reducing the risk of scarring and infection. This property is particularly beneficial for aging skin, which often heals more slowly due to reduced cell turnover.

2. Improved Muscle Recovery and Physical Resilience

For athletes and active individuals, Thymosin Beta-4 is highly valued for its ability to support muscle recovery. By reducing inflammation and promoting cell migration, TB4 helps repair microtears in muscles, allowing for faster recovery after intense workouts. This benefit extends to those dealing with muscle strain or injury, making TB4 a versatile aid for maintaining physical resilience.

3. Joint and Tendon Support

Joint and tendon health is essential for mobility and quality of life, especially as we age. Thymosin Beta-4 supports the health of these connective tissues by promoting collagen production and reducing inflammation, which helps maintain flexibility, reduce pain, and protect against strain or injury.

4. Strengthened Immune System

A healthy immune system is crucial for defending against infections and illnesses, particularly in later years. Thymosin Beta-4 enhances immune function by supporting T-cell activity and moderating inflammatory responses. This immune support reduces the risk of infections and provides added resilience against chronic inflammation, which can accelerate aging.

5. Enhanced Skin Health and Elasticity

As a peptide that promotes collagen synthesis and cellular migration, Thymosin Beta-4 is beneficial for skin health. Collagen is a vital protein that keeps skin firm, smooth, and elastic, but its production declines with age. TB4 helps replenish collagen levels, reducing the appearance of wrinkles, improving elasticity, and supporting a youthful complexion.

Using Thymosin Beta-4 in a Health Routine

Integrating Thymosin Beta-4 into a health routine can provide valuable support for immunity, recovery, and overall wellness. While TB4 is commonly administered via injection for systemic effects, topical and oral forms are also becoming available, particularly for localized or digestive benefits.

1. Injectable Thymosin Beta-4

Injectable TB4 is the most effective method for delivering this peptide to the bloodstream, allowing it to reach various tissues throughout the body. Injections can be administered subcutaneously or intramuscularly, depending on the area of focus. Consulting a healthcare provider for guidance on dosage and administration is recommended, especially for those new to peptide therapy.

2. Topical Thymosin Beta-4

For those interested in skin or localized healing, TB4 is available in topical formulations, such as creams or gels, that can be applied directly to the skin. This method is ideal for targeting specific areas, such as wounds, scars, or areas of inflammation.

3. Oral Thymosin Beta-4

Oral TB4 supplements are less common but can be useful for supporting digestive health or providing systemic immune support. While oral TB4 may not be as potent as injections, it offers a convenient alternative for those who prefer non-invasive methods.

Potential Side Effects and Safety of Thymosin Beta-4

Thymosin Beta-4 is generally well-tolerated when used appropriately, with few reported side effects. Some individuals may experience mild irritation at the injection site or, in rare cases, temporary symptoms such as fatigue or digestive discomfort. These side effects are typically mild and resolve on their own.

To ensure safety, it is important to follow recommended dosages and consult a healthcare provider before beginning TB4 therapy. As with any peptide treatment, professional guidance is key to achieving optimal results while minimizing potential risks.

The Future of Thymosin Beta-4 in Medicine and Wellness

The therapeutic potential of Thymosin Beta-4 continues to be explored, with research delving into its possible applications for autoimmune conditions, heart health, and even neurodegenerative diseases. As science advances, Thymosin Beta-4's role in medicine may expand, particularly in regenerative therapies that aim to harness the body's own healing capabilities.

In the context of anti-aging and wellness, Thymosin Beta-4 represents a promising path forward. Its ability to support immune health, accelerate recovery, and promote tissue repair aligns well with the goals of those seeking to age with resilience and vitality. Whether used alone or in combination with other peptides, Thymosin Beta-4 offers a versatile approach to maintaining health, activity, and quality of life.

2.5 CJC-1295 and Ipamorelin – Growth Hormone Boosters

As we age, the natural production of growth hormone—one of the body's critical regulators of metabolism, muscle growth, and cellular repair—begins to decline. This decline is often linked to a host of aging signs, including decreased muscle mass, slower recovery times, reduced energy levels, and changes in body composition. In the search for solutions to slow this process and promote a more youthful vitality, two peptides have gained considerable attention for their unique synergy and effectiveness in stimulating growth hormone release: CJC-1295 and Ipamorelin.

CJC-1295 and Ipamorelin are commonly used together because they each target growth hormone production in complementary ways, amplifying the effects and supporting a broad range of health and anti-aging benefits. Together, they work by signaling the pituitary gland to release growth hormone in a way that mimics the body's natural rhythms, allowing for controlled and sustained release rather than abrupt spikes. This gentle yet effective stimulation of growth hormone levels makes the CJC-1295 and Ipamorelin combination a popular choice among those seeking to improve muscle tone, increase energy, enhance recovery, and enjoy the restorative effects associated with growth hormone.

What are CJC-1295 and Ipamorelin?

CJC-1295 and Ipamorelin are peptides that each play a role in the regulation of growth hormone, but they work in slightly different ways. CJC-1295 is a growth hormone-releasing hormone (GHRH) analog, which means it acts on the pituitary gland to stimulate the release of growth hormone. Its structure is designed to bind to receptors on the pituitary gland, encouraging the production of growth hormone in a controlled, sustained manner. CJC-1295's effects last longer due to its extended half-life, allowing it to stimulate growth hormone production over a prolonged period.

Ipamorelin, on the other hand, is a growth hormone-releasing peptide (GHRP). It works by stimulating the release of growth hormone-releasing factors from the hypothalamus, a region in the brain that regulates numerous bodily functions, including metabolism and growth. Ipamorelin is unique among GHRPs because it is highly selective for growth hormone and does not raise levels of cortisol or prolactin, which can have unwanted side effects. This selectivity makes Ipamorelin particularly attractive for those looking for the benefits of increased growth hormone without the risk of hormonal imbalances.

When used together, CJC-1295 and Ipamorelin complement each other, creating a synergistic effect that enhances the body's natural ability to release growth hormone. By combining a GHRH analog with a GHRP, this duo can increase growth hormone levels more effectively than either peptide could on its own, while closely mimicking the body's natural growth hormone release patterns.

How CJC-1295 and Ipamorelin Work: The Science of Growth Hormone Stimulation

The human body relies on growth hormone for numerous functions, from tissue repair and metabolism regulation to muscle and bone maintenance. Growth hormone is released in pulses, with levels peaking during deep sleep and tapering off during the day. This natural pulsatile release helps the body maintain balance, supporting energy, recovery, and overall health without overwhelming the system. As we age, however, these pulses become smaller and less frequent, contributing to the signs of aging.

The CJC-1295 and Ipamorelin combination works by encouraging these growth hormone pulses, helping to restore a pattern closer to what is seen in younger individuals. Here's a closer look at how each peptide contributes to this process:

1. CJC-1295 and Sustained Growth Hormone Release

CJC-1295 is designed to extend the period during which growth hormone is released. This peptide binds to receptors on the pituitary gland and encourages growth hormone production in a controlled, sustained manner. With a longer half-life than many other GHRH analogs, CJC-1295 provides a steady stimulation, allowing for more consistent growth hormone release and ensuring that growth hormone levels remain elevated for a longer period.

2. Ipamorelin and Pulsatile Growth Hormone Secretion

Ipamorelin complements CJC-1295 by stimulating the release of growth hormone from the hypothalamus, which controls the body's natural hormonal rhythms. Ipamorelin is particularly effective at initiating growth hormone pulses without affecting cortisol or prolactin, which helps prevent the potential side effects associated with other GHRPs. This pulsatile effect mirrors the body's natural growth hormone release, enhancing the benefits without disrupting hormonal balance.

3. Synergy Between CJC-1295 and Ipamorelin

Together, CJC-1295 and Ipamorelin create a balanced approach to growth hormone stimulation. CJC-1295 provides a sustained release, while Ipamorelin promotes pulsatile secretion, ensuring that growth hormone is available when the body needs it most—such as during sleep or recovery periods. This combination is designed to mimic the natural rhythms of growth hormone release, which supports a wide range of physiological processes that are crucial for anti-aging and health.

Benefits of CJC-1295 and Ipamorelin for Anti-Aging and Wellness

The increase in growth hormone levels brought about by CJC-1295 and Ipamorelin can yield numerous benefits for health, wellness, and longevity. Here are some of the key advantages that users may experience:

1. Enhanced Muscle Growth and Recovery
Growth hormone plays a significant role in muscle protein synthesis, which is essential for building and repairing muscle tissue. With higher growth hormone levels, the body can more effectively repair muscle fibers after exercise, promoting muscle growth and reducing recovery time. This benefit is especially valuable for athletes and those who engage in regular physical activity, as it allows for more frequent and effective workouts.

2. Improved Body Composition

Growth hormone influences body composition by promoting fat metabolism and supporting lean muscle development. Higher growth hormone levels can increase the body's ability to burn fat, particularly around the abdomen, while preserving muscle mass. This shift in body composition contributes to a leaner, more toned physique, making it easier to maintain a healthy weight and appearance as we age.

3. Increased Energy and Vitality

Many people report feeling more energetic and youthful when growth hormone levels are optimized. Growth hormone supports cellular energy production, which translates to better stamina, higher energy levels, and a greater capacity to engage in daily activities. The energy boost provided by CJC-1295 and Ipamorelin can help combat age-related fatigue, allowing individuals to remain active and engaged.

4. Better Sleep Quality and Recovery

Growth hormone release peaks during deep sleep, which is crucial for the body's repair and recovery processes. By supporting growth hormone levels, CJC-1295 and Ipamorelin can enhance sleep quality, allowing for more restorative rest. This improvement in sleep quality not only supports physical recovery but also promotes mental clarity, mood stability, and resilience against stress.

5. Enhanced Skin Health and Elasticity

Growth hormone is associated with collagen synthesis, which plays a vital role in maintaining skin elasticity and firmness. By stimulating growth hormone release, CJC-1295 and Ipamorelin can support the skin's natural regeneration processes, reducing the appearance of fine lines and wrinkles. This improvement in skin health contributes to a more youthful appearance and supports long-term skin integrity.

6. Strengthened Immune System

Growth hormone supports immune cell function, helping the body defend against infections and illnesses. By enhancing growth hormone levels, CJC-1295 and Ipamorelin may provide immune support, making it easier for the body to fend off pathogens and recover from illness.

Using CJC-1295 and Ipamorelin in a Wellness Routine

The CJC-1295 and Ipamorelin combination is most commonly administered through subcutaneous injections, allowing the peptides to be absorbed directly into the bloodstream for effective results. This approach maximizes bioavailability and ensures that the peptides can act efficiently on the pituitary gland and hypothalamus.

1. Dosage and Administration

CJC-1295 and Ipamorelin are typically administered together in a single injection, either once or twice daily. Doses and frequency depend on individual health goals, age, and lifestyle, so it's essential to consult a healthcare provider who can tailor a regimen to your specific needs. Many users choose to inject the combination before bedtime to take advantage of the body's natural growth hormone release during sleep.

2. Maintaining a Healthy Lifestyle

While CJC-1295 and Ipamorelin can support growth hormone levels, maintaining a healthy lifestyle is crucial for maximizing the benefits. Regular exercise, a balanced diet, quality sleep, and stress management all contribute to overall well-being and amplify the effects of growth hormone optimization. By combining these peptides with healthy habits, users can achieve a more comprehensive approach to anti-aging and wellness.

3. Monitoring and Adjusting

Regular health check-ups and monitoring can help assess how well the peptides are working and whether any adjustments to the dosage or schedule are necessary. Blood tests can help track growth hormone levels, body composition, and other markers of health, ensuring that the treatment remains effective and safe.

Potential Side Effects and Safety of CJC-1295 and Ipamorelin

CJC-1295 and Ipamorelin are generally well-tolerated, especially when used under the guidance of a healthcare provider. However, as with any peptide treatment, some individuals may experience mild side effects, such as temporary nausea, headaches, or slight irritation at the injection site. These side effects are usually minimal and tend to resolve quickly.

To minimize risks, it's essential to follow recommended dosages and consult with a healthcare provider before starting treatment. Regular monitoring can help ensure that the treatment is working as intended without causing unwanted side effects.

The Future of Growth Hormone Boosters in Anti-Aging Science

As research into peptides and growth hormone modulation advances, we may see more refined and personalized approaches to growth hormone optimization. Scientists are exploring how peptides like CJC-1295 and Ipamorelin can be combined with other therapies, such as lifestyle interventions and complementary peptides, to create comprehensive anti-aging programs.

With their potential to support muscle growth, fat metabolism, immune health, and recovery, CJC-1295 and Ipamorelin represent an exciting frontier in the science of longevity. By enhancing the body's natural rhythms and supporting growth hormone levels, these peptides offer a promising option for those seeking to age with energy, resilience, and vitality.

2.6   Selecting   Peptides   for   Your Anti-Aging Goals

With the vast array of peptides available for anti-aging, selecting the right ones for your personal goals can seem overwhelming. Each peptide offers unique benefits, targeting specific aspects of aging such as skin health, muscle preservation, cognitive function, or immune support. Whether you're looking to maintain a youthful complexion, increase vitality, or promote recovery and resilience, understanding how to choose the right peptides is essential for maximizing results.

Defining Your Anti-Aging Goals

Before diving into specific peptides, it's helpful to define what "anti-aging" means for you personally. While anti-aging may conjure images of smoother skin or fewer wrinkles, the term encompasses a wide range of health and wellness goals. These can include physical resilience, cognitive sharpness, hormonal balance, immune support, and much more. By identifying your primary focus, you can streamline the peptide selection process to ensure you're targeting the areas most important to you.

1. Skin Health and Appearance

For those focused on skin rejuvenation, peptides like GHK-Cu are highly effective in promoting collagen synthesis, improving elasticity, and enhancing skin hydration. Other peptides, such as Thymosin Beta-4, can support healing and reduce inflammation, which is beneficial for maintaining a youthful complexion.

2. Physical Recovery and Muscle Preservation

If muscle health, recovery, and physical resilience are priorities, growth hormone-boosting peptides like CJC-1295 and Ipamorelin can be valuable. These peptides help stimulate growth hormone release, which supports muscle repair and fat metabolism. BPC-157, known for its healing properties, is another good choice for promoting joint and tendon health.

3. Longevity and Cellular Health

Those focused on overall longevity and cellular health may benefit from peptides like Epitalon, which supports telomere length and has shown potential in promoting longevity at a cellular level. Thymosin Beta-4, with its immune-boosting and regenerative properties, also contributes to healthier aging and can be an excellent addition for long-term wellness.

4. Cognitive Function and Mental Clarity

For cognitive support, certain peptides known for promoting brain health and neuroprotection are beneficial. While peptides like CJC-1295 indirectly support mental health by improving sleep and recovery, others, such as those being studied for neuroprotective effects, can be included to support mental clarity and focus.

5. Immune Support and Inflammation Control

If immune health is a focus, Thymosin Beta-4 is particularly effective, as it supports immune cell activity and helps reduce inflammation. Peptides that promote recovery, reduce inflammation, and support immune balance can contribute to better resilience against infections and illnesses.

Key Peptides for Different Anti-Aging Goals

Let's break down some of the most popular peptides and how they align with specific anti-aging goals. By understanding their primary functions and effects, you'll be able to select the ones best suited to your needs.

1. GHK-Cu for Skin Rejuvenation

GHK-Cu is often called the "skin rejuvenator" due to its ability to promote collagen synthesis, improve skin elasticity, and support wound healing. It is an excellent choice for those focused on enhancing skin appearance, reducing wrinkles, and achieving a radiant complexion. GHK-Cu's antioxidant properties also make it beneficial for reducing oxidative stress, a common contributor to skin aging.

2. BPC-157 for Physical Recovery and Joint Health

Known as the "healing peptide," BPC-157 is renowned for its ability to promote tissue repair, reduce inflammation, and support joint and tendon health. This peptide is highly recommended for athletes, active individuals, or anyone dealing with physical strain, as it enhances recovery and resilience against injury. BPC-157 can be used alone or in combination with growth hormone-stimulating peptides like CJC-1295 and Ipamorelin for comprehensive physical support.

3. Epitalon for Longevity and Cellular Health

Epitalon, often called the "longevity enhancer," activates telomerase production, which helps maintain telomere length and promotes cellular health. Epitalon is a good choice for those interested in supporting long-term health and potentially extending their lifespan. By preserving telomeres, Epitalon helps cells remain functional for longer, which is beneficial for aging at the cellular level.

**4. CJC-1295 and Ipamorelin for Muscle Preservation and
Metabolic Health**

This peptide duo is ideal for individuals focused on
maintaining muscle mass, supporting fat metabolism, and
improving energy levels. CJC-1295 and Ipamorelin stimulate
growth hormone release, which helps support muscle
recovery, maintain lean body mass, and improve metabolic
efficiency. This combination is popular among those looking
to maintain physical vitality and resilience as they age.

5. Thymosin Beta-4 for Immunity and Resilience

Thymosin Beta-4 (TB4) is known for its
immune-modulating properties and its ability to reduce
inflammation. It helps regulate immune cell activity, supports
wound healing, and enhances tissue regeneration. TB4 is
beneficial for those focused on maintaining a strong immune
system, particularly as they age, making it a good choice for
supporting overall wellness and resilience.

Creating a Personalized Peptide Stack

For those with multiple anti-aging goals, creating a peptide
stack—a combination of peptides that work well
together—can be an effective way to achieve comprehensive
results. Stacking peptides allows you to address different
aspects of aging simultaneously, such as skin health, muscle
preservation, and immune support.

When creating a stack, it's essential to consider how each
peptide works individually and how they complement each
other. Here are some examples of peptide stacks based on
common anti-aging goals:

1. Skin Health Stack
GHK-Cu: Supports collagen synthesis, skin elasticity, and wound healing.
Thymosin Beta-4: Reduces inflammation and promotes skin repair.
This combination targets skin health from both a structural and inflammatory perspective, providing a balanced approach to maintaining youthful skin.

2. Muscle and Recovery Stack
CJC-1295 and Ipamorelin: Boost growth hormone levels for muscle growth and recovery.
BPC-157: Promotes healing and reduces inflammation in muscles, joints, and tendons.
Together, these peptides provide a comprehensive approach to muscle recovery and joint health, ideal for those with active lifestyles.

3. Longevity and Cellular Health Stack
Epitalon: Supports telomere length and cellular health.
Thymosin Beta-4: Enhances immune function and promotes tissue regeneration.
This stack supports long-term health by focusing on cellular preservation and immune resilience, helping to maintain vitality and reduce age-related decline.

4. Immune Support Stack
Thymosin Beta-4: Regulates immune cell activity and reduces inflammation.

GHK-Cu: Provides antioxidant support to reduce oxidative stress.

By combining immune support and antioxidant protection, this stack enhances the body's defenses against infections and reduces chronic inflammation.

Integrating Peptides Into Your Routine

Once you've selected peptides that align with your anti-aging goals, it's essential to incorporate them into your routine in a way that maximizes their effectiveness. Here are some tips for using peptides effectively:

1. Follow Recommended Dosages

Each peptide has its specific dosage range and recommended administration frequency. Following these guidelines ensures that you receive the desired benefits without the risk of overuse or side effects. Consult a healthcare provider with experience in peptide therapy to determine the appropriate dosages for your individual needs.

2. Consider Timing and Frequency

Some peptides are most effective when taken at specific times. For example, growth hormone-releasing peptides like CJC-1295 and Ipamorelin are often taken before bedtime to coincide with the body's natural growth hormone release during deep sleep. Thymosin Beta-4 and BPC-157 may be administered in the morning or post-exercise for optimal recovery support.

3. Maintain Consistency

Like most wellness practices, consistency is key to achieving the best results with peptides. Use the peptides regularly according to the recommended schedule, as results often take time to become noticeable. A consistent routine helps maximize the cumulative effects, particularly for peptides involved in tissue repair and cellular health.

4. Combine With a Healthy Lifestyle

Peptides work best when paired with healthy lifestyle habits. A balanced diet, regular exercise, quality sleep, and stress management are all essential for supporting anti-aging goals. These habits complement the effects of peptides and help create a foundation for long-term health and vitality.

5. Monitor Progress and Adjust as Needed

Regular check-ups and monitoring can help assess the effectiveness of your peptide regimen and determine if adjustments are needed. Blood tests, health markers, and even physical changes can provide valuable feedback, allowing you to fine-tune your approach over time.

Safety Considerations When Selecting Peptides

While peptides are generally well-tolerated, it's important to use them safely and responsibly. Working with a healthcare provider ensures that you are using the right peptides, dosages, and protocols for your needs. Additionally, only purchase peptides from reputable sources to avoid low-quality products that may be ineffective or unsafe.

Building a Personalized Anti-Aging Peptide Routine

Selecting peptides for anti-aging is about more than just choosing the "best" ones; it's about creating a routine tailored to your unique goals, lifestyle, and health priorities. Whether your focus is on skin health, muscle recovery, immune support, or longevity, peptides offer powerful tools to help you achieve and maintain vitality.

As you begin your peptide journey, remember that patience and consistency are key. With the right approach, peptides can enhance your body's natural regenerative abilities, providing a pathway to aging gracefully and maintaining wellness at every stage of life.

Chapter 3: Protocols and Peptide Stacking for Optimal Results

3.1 Safe Dosage and Application Methods

Embarking on a journey with peptides for anti-aging and wellness requires a clear understanding of safe dosage and proper application methods. Peptides are powerful tools that can support everything from skin health and muscle recovery to immune function and longevity, but they must be used responsibly to ensure safety and effectiveness. Safe usage depends on selecting the right dose, understanding administration techniques, and following protocols tailored to individual needs.

Understanding Dosage: Why It Matters

One of the most important aspects of peptide therapy is getting the dosage right. Too little may result in limited benefits, while too much can increase the risk of side effects or disrupt your body's natural balance. Finding the optimal dosage involves considering factors such as your age, health goals, weight, and overall wellness. Peptide dosages are typically measured in micrograms (mcg) or milligrams (mg), and each peptide has its own recommended range based on its purpose and potency.

Since peptide therapy is still an emerging field, it's best to work with a healthcare provider experienced in peptide therapy to determine the right dosage for you. This professional guidance can help you avoid overuse or underuse and ensure that you're receiving the maximum benefits safely.

General Guidelines for Safe Peptide Dosage

Although individual needs vary, there are general guidelines for dosing that can serve as a starting point. Below is an overview of recommended dosages for some popular peptides, but remember that these are typical ranges and may need to be adjusted based on your specific situation.

1. GHK-Cu (Copper Peptide)
- **Common Dosage:** 1-2 mg per application, applied once or twice daily for topical use; 100-200 mcg daily for subcutaneous injections.
- **Purpose:** Skin health, collagen synthesis, antioxidant support.

- **Guidance:** GHK-Cu is commonly used as a topical serum or cream for skin benefits. When used in injections, it should be kept within the recommended range to avoid skin sensitivity.

2. BPC-157

- **Common Dosage:** 200-500 mcg per injection, one to two times daily.
- **Purpose:** Tissue repair, inflammation reduction, joint and tendon support.
- **Guidance:** BPC-157 is frequently used for muscle recovery and joint health. It's essential to stick to lower doses initially and adjust as needed, especially when treating specific injuries.

3. Epitalon

- **Common Dosage:** 5-10 mg per injection, administered over a cycle (e.g., once daily for 10-20 days).
- **Purpose:** Telomere maintenance, longevity support, immune enhancement.
- **Guidance:** Epitalon is often used in cycles to maximize its longevity benefits. Taking breaks between cycles is recommended to avoid overuse.

4. CJC-1295 with Ipamorelin

- **Common Dosage:** 100-200 mcg of each peptide per injection, typically taken once daily (often before bedtime).
- **Purpose:** Growth hormone release, muscle preservation, fat metabolism.

- **Guidance:** This combination is popular for its synergistic effects on growth hormone stimulation. Dosages are often started on the lower end and gradually increased as needed.

5. Thymosin Beta-4 (TB4)
- **Common Dosage:** 2-5 mg per injection, administered weekly.
- **Purpose:** Immune support, tissue regeneration, anti-inflammatory effects.
- **Guidance:** Thymosin Beta-4 is typically used in periodic doses, depending on the specific health goals, to support healing and immunity.

Application Methods: Choosing the Right Approach

Peptides can be administered in several ways, each with its own advantages and best-use scenarios. The most common methods are injections, topical application, and oral supplementation. Understanding these methods will help you choose the approach that aligns with your goals and comfort level.

1. Injectable Peptides

Injectable peptides are the most common and effective method for peptide administration, as they allow peptides to enter the bloodstream directly, bypassing digestion and ensuring high bioavailability. Injection types include subcutaneous (under the skin) and intramuscular (into the muscle), both of which are commonly used depending on the peptide and target area.

- **Subcutaneous Injections:**

Subcutaneous injections involve injecting peptides just beneath the skin, typically into fatty tissue areas such as the abdomen or thigh. This method is suitable for peptides like BPC-157, CJC-1295, and Ipamorelin and is generally easy for self-administration with proper guidance. A fine, short needle is used, and the process is relatively painless.

- **Intramuscular Injections:**

Intramuscular injections are delivered into the muscle, allowing for faster absorption in some cases. This method may be used for specific peptides that benefit from rapid uptake. However, intramuscular injections require more precision and are usually administered by a healthcare provider or with thorough instruction.

2. Topical Peptides

Topical application is a non-invasive method best suited for peptides aimed at skin health, such as GHK-Cu. Topical peptides are formulated as creams, serums, or gels and are applied directly to the skin. This method is ideal for those focused on improving skin tone, elasticity, and hydration, as it allows peptides to target the dermal layers without systemic absorption.

Application Tips

For maximum absorption, cleanse your skin before applying a peptide serum or cream. Gently massage the product into the skin, allowing it to fully absorb before applying other products. Use as directed, typically once or twice daily.

3. Oral Peptides

While less common, some peptides are available in oral form, typically as capsules or tablets. This method is convenient and user-friendly, especially for peptides aimed at gastrointestinal health, such as BPC-157. However, oral peptides may have lower bioavailability, as they must pass through the digestive system before being absorbed. As a result, injectable forms are generally preferred for systemic benefits.

Considerations:

If you choose oral peptides, be aware that they may have a slower onset of effects. They are generally used for more localized or digestive benefits rather than broad-spectrum anti-aging purposes.

Safe Administration Practices

Administering peptides safely involves using proper techniques, storing peptides correctly, and following hygiene practices to prevent contamination or infection. Here are some tips for safe peptide administration:

1. Practice Proper Injection Technique

If using injectable peptides, ensure you're using the correct technique, including needle size, injection depth, and site rotation. Always use a sterile needle for each injection and follow a step-by-step process to avoid accidental injury or infection. Many people choose to work with a healthcare provider initially to learn proper techniques before self-administration.

2. Rotate Injection Sites

To minimize discomfort and prevent tissue irritation, rotate your injection sites. This is particularly important for daily injections, such as those used with CJC-1295 and Ipamorelin. Common sites include the abdomen, thigh, and upper arm.

3. Store Peptides Properly

Peptides should be stored according to the manufacturer's instructions, often in a refrigerator to maintain stability. Exposure to heat or light can degrade peptides, reducing their effectiveness. For injectable peptides, only mix with sterile water immediately before use to maintain potency.

4. Maintain Hygiene and Sterility

Always wash your hands and disinfect the injection area with alcohol before administering peptides. Use alcohol wipes on vials, needles, and skin to prevent contamination. Dispose of needles safely in a designated sharps container.

Monitoring Results and Adjusting Dosage

Since peptide therapy works over time, tracking your progress and being attentive to any changes in your body is essential. Keeping a journal of your dosages, application times, and observed effects can be helpful in assessing the effectiveness of your regimen. Regular check-ups and blood tests can provide valuable insight, helping you adjust your protocol if necessary.

Starting Low and Adjusting Gradually:

Many users begin with lower doses to gauge how their body responds, then gradually increase dosage as needed. This approach reduces the likelihood of side effects and allows you to fine-tune the dose for optimal results.

Consulting with a Healthcare Provider:
Professional guidance is crucial for determining when and how to adjust dosages, particularly with peptides that affect hormone levels, such as CJC-1295 and Ipamorelin. Regular consultations help ensure you're receiving the right amount for your goals while monitoring any health markers that may require attention.

Potential Side Effects and Safety Considerations

Peptides are generally safe when used within recommended dosages, but side effects can still occur, particularly if dosages are too high or the body is sensitive to specific peptides. Common side effects include mild irritation at the injection site, fatigue, nausea, and, in some cases, headaches.

To minimize risks, adhere to these safety guidelines:

1. Stay Within Recommended Dosages:
 Avoid exceeding the recommended dosage ranges for each peptide, as overuse can increase the risk of side effects. Sticking to conservative dosages can provide steady benefits without overwhelming the body.

2. Monitor for Unusual Symptoms:
 If you experience any symptoms beyond mild side effects, such as persistent nausea, dizziness, or unexpected hormonal changes, discontinue use and consult a healthcare provider.

3. Ensure Product Quality:
Only purchase peptides from reputable sources that adhere to quality standards. Low-quality peptides may contain impurities or inactive ingredients, which can compromise safety and efficacy.

Building a Safe and Effective Peptide Routine

Integrating peptides into your wellness routine requires attention to detail, from selecting the right dosage and application method to monitoring progress and making adjustments as needed. By prioritizing safety and following recommended practices, you can unlock the potential of peptides for anti-aging, recovery, and overall health in a way that supports your long-term goals.

3.2 Peptide Stacks and Their Benefits

As the field of peptide therapy expands, so does the understanding of how different peptides can be combined, or **"stacked,"** to enhance their benefits. Peptide stacking involves using two or more peptides in tandem to address multiple aspects of health and aging simultaneously. For instance, a combination that promotes both muscle recovery and skin elasticity can provide comprehensive anti-aging support. Each peptide in a stack has a unique mechanism, and when chosen carefully, they work synergistically to create a more robust and effective outcome.

What is Peptide Stacking?

Peptide stacking is the process of combining different peptides to maximize benefits and target specific health outcomes more effectively. Stacks can be as simple as pairing two peptides or more complex, involving multiple peptides that address various aspects of aging, such as skin health, muscle support, and immune function.

When stacking peptides, it's important to select those that complement each other without causing overstimulation. For example, a stack focused on growth hormone optimization may include CJC-1295 and Ipamorelin, both of which stimulate growth hormone release but through different mechanisms. This complementary action enhances the effects without overloading the body.

Choosing the right stack depends on your goals, lifestyle, and tolerance, and it's advisable to consult a healthcare provider to ensure that your stack is balanced and safe.

Tips for Stacking Peptides Effectively

1. Start with a Single Stack:
If you're new to peptide therapy, start with one stack to assess how your body responds before adding additional peptides.

This approach helps you gauge effectiveness and avoid potential side effects.

2. Cycle Peptides as Needed:

Some peptides, such as Epitalon, are most effective when used in cycles to prevent overstimulation. Follow recommended cycle protocols to give your body time to adjust and benefit from each peptide.

3. Consult a Healthcare Provider:

Combining peptides requires careful consideration of dosages and timing. A healthcare provider experienced in peptide therapy can help you design a safe, effective stack based on your individual goals and health profile.

4. Monitor Progress and Adjust Accordingly:

Keep track of your results and how you feel while using a peptide stack. Adjust dosages, timing, or individual peptides as needed to optimize your outcomes.

5. Prioritize Quality and Consistency:

Only purchase peptides from reputable sources, and use them consistently according to protocol. Proper storage and administration are essential for maintaining peptide effectiveness.

Creating Your Ideal Peptide Stack

Peptide stacking is a powerful tool for addressing multiple aspects of aging and health, allowing you to create a tailored approach that aligns with your goals. By carefully selecting peptides that complement each other, you can support everything from skin health and muscle recovery to immune function and cellular longevity.

3.3 Peptide Programs for Beginners, Intermediate, and Advanced Users

Starting a peptide regimen can feel daunting for new users, while those with experience may be looking for more advanced protocols to maximize their benefits. Structuring a peptide program based on your experience level—whether you're a beginner, intermediate, or advanced user—can help you integrate peptides into your wellness routine more effectively. Each level builds upon the last, allowing users to explore peptides at a comfortable pace, ensuring safe, consistent progress.

Beginner Peptide Program: A Gentle Introduction

For beginners, the focus should be on simplicity and safety, using peptides that offer clear, manageable benefits with minimal side effects. This level is ideal for users new to peptide therapy who want to observe how peptides affect their body without introducing complexity. The goal is to establish a solid foundation, learning proper dosages, application methods, and best practices.

Primary Goals for Beginners:
- Introduce peptides in a low-dose, easy-to-manage regimen.
- Focus on visible, short-term benefits (e.g., improved skin health, slight boost in recovery).
- Build familiarity with peptide applications and observe the body's responses.

Recommended Peptides and Protocols

1. GHK-Cu for Skin Health and Anti-Aging
Dosage: 1-2 mg applied topically, once daily.
Application: Apply as a serum or cream to the face and neck area to improve skin elasticity, tone, and hydration.
Benefits: This peptide is widely recognized for its ability to promote collagen production, improve skin firmness, and provide antioxidant protection. It's an ideal starting point for those interested in visible anti-aging benefits without injections.

2. BPC-157 for Recovery and Inflammation
Dosage: 200 mcg per day, injected subcutaneously (near injury sites if applicable).
Application: BPC-157 can be injected under the skin or administered orally, making it versatile for users comfortable with either method.
Benefits: Known as the **"healing peptide,"** BPC-157 supports joint health, accelerates tissue repair, and reduces inflammation. It's a practical choice for beginners experiencing muscle soreness or inflammation from exercise or daily activities.

3. Basic Program Overview:
Schedule: GHK-Cu is used daily, while BPC-157 can be used as needed or in cycles (e.g., daily for two weeks, then a break).
Goals: This program targets skin health and muscle recovery, providing an easy entry into peptide therapy with visible, accessible benefits.

Intermediate Peptide Program: Building on Basics

For those who have some experience with peptides and feel comfortable with self-administration, the intermediate program adds new peptides with complementary effects to create a balanced stack. At this stage, the focus expands to include more complex goals, such as muscle preservation, immune support, and moderate anti-aging effects. Intermediate users may be ready to use multiple peptides simultaneously, combining topical and injectable peptides in a well-rounded routine.

Primary Goals for Intermediate Users:
- Introduce additional peptides with complementary benefits.
- Address multiple health goals (e.g., muscle support, immune function, skin health).
- Start using peptide combinations (stacking) for more comprehensive results.

Recommended Peptides and Protocols:

1. CJC-1295 and Ipamorelin for Growth Hormone Release

Dosage: 100-200 mcg of each peptide per day, injected subcutaneously before bedtime.

Application: Inject CJC-1295 and Ipamorelin together to optimize growth hormone release during sleep.

Benefits: This peptide duo is known for its effects on growth hormone, supporting muscle growth, fat metabolism, and recovery. It's a popular choice for those looking to maintain lean muscle and improve energy levels.

2. Thymosin Beta-4 for Immune Support and Recovery

Dosage: 2-5 mg per week, administered subcutaneously.

Application: TB4 injections can be given weekly, supporting immune function and reducing inflammation.

Benefits: TB4 promotes tissue repair, supports immune health, and helps manage inflammation, making it suitable for individuals focused on resilience and recovery.

3. Intermediate Program Overview:

Schedule: CJC-1295 and Ipamorelin are administered daily, while Thymosin Beta-4 is used weekly. This stack can be used for 4-6 weeks, followed by a break.

Goals: This program combines growth hormone stimulation, immune support, and anti-inflammatory effects, enhancing muscle tone, recovery, and overall resilience.

Advanced Peptide Program: Comprehensive Stacking for Multi-Faceted Benefits

Advanced users often have extensive experience with peptide therapy and are comfortable managing multiple peptides and injection routines. The advanced program introduces more specialized peptides, allowing users to address various aspects of aging, recovery, metabolism, and cognitive health. At this level, the program is highly customizable, with tailored peptide stacks that can be adjusted based on specific goals and health markers.

Primary Goals for Advanced Users:
- Utilize specialized peptides targeting diverse health aspects.
- Fine-tune peptide combinations (complex stacking) for maximum synergy.
- Focus on long-term anti-aging, cognitive enhancement, and immune resilience.

Recommended Peptides and Protocols:

1. Epitalon for Longevity and Cellular Health
Dosage: 5-10 mg per day, injected subcutaneously for 10-20 days in a cycle, followed by a break.
Application: Epitalon is administered in cycles to stimulate telomerase and support cellular longevity.
Benefits: Epitalon is known for its ability to activate telomerase, preserving telomere length and supporting long-term cellular health. It's ideal for those focused on longevity and aging prevention.

2. CJC-1295 and Ipamorelin for Muscle and Metabolic Health
Dosage: 200 mcg of each peptide per day, injected subcutaneously.
Application: This combination is best administered at night, aligning with the body's growth hormone release during sleep.

Benefits: This stack continues to support growth hormone production, promoting muscle preservation, metabolism, and energy levels.

3. MOTS-c for Metabolic Health and Energy
Dosage: 5 mg per injection, taken 1-3 times per week.
Application: MOTS-c can be injected to enhance mitochondrial function and support metabolic health.
Benefits: MOTS-c is a mitochondrial peptide that enhances glucose metabolism, supporting energy and promoting a healthy body composition. It's an advanced peptide for those interested in metabolic health.

4. Advanced Program Overview:
Schedule: Epitalon is used in cycles, CJC-1295 and Ipamorelin are taken daily, and MOTS-c is injected weekly or as needed. Advanced users can customize this regimen based on specific health metrics and long-term goals.
Goals: This program combines cellular longevity, growth hormone stimulation, and metabolic support, offering a comprehensive anti-aging approach.

3.4   Sample   Usage   Protocols   and Monitoring Progress

Starting a peptide routine is an exciting journey, but it's essential to have a structured plan to make the most of the peptides you're using. Sample usage protocols serve as helpful guides, illustrating how peptides can be scheduled and cycled to achieve specific health goals, from muscle growth and recovery to skin rejuvenation and immune support. Alongside these protocols, tracking your progress is key to understanding how well your regimen is working and making adjustments as needed.

Monitoring Progress: Keeping Track of Your Results

Monitoring your progress is a critical aspect of a successful peptide regimen. Observing how your body responds over time helps ensure that you're getting the most out of your protocol and allows for any necessary adjustments. Here are some practical tips for tracking and evaluating your results.

1. Keep a Journal
Recording your experience in a health journal can provide valuable insights into how peptides are affecting your body. In your journal, note the following:

Dosages and Timing: Record which peptides you're using, the dosages, and when you administer them.
Physical Observations: Document changes in energy levels, muscle recovery times, skin texture, or joint pain.
Overall Wellness: Track any changes in sleep quality, immune resilience, or mental clarity.
Mood and Energy: Some peptides can impact mood and vitality, so noting any psychological changes can be helpful.

2. Use Before and After Photos

For goals related to physical appearance, such as skin health or muscle growth, before and after photos can be incredibly informative. Photos provide a visual record of changes, helping you assess progress with greater accuracy.

Skin Health: Take close-up photos of specific areas you're targeting, like the face or neck, under consistent lighting.
Muscle Tone: For muscle growth protocols, capture full-body photos, ideally at the same time of day to ensure consistency.

3. Track Workouts and Recovery

For those using peptides to enhance muscle growth and recovery, keeping a log of your workouts is invaluable. Document your workout intensity, any muscle soreness, and your recovery times.

Exercise Performance: Note changes in strength, endurance, and workout intensity.
Recovery Times: Record how quickly you recover from strenuous workouts or physical exertion, as peptides often reduce recovery time.

4. Schedule Regular Check-Ups and Blood Tests

For advanced protocols, especially those affecting hormones or metabolic markers, consider scheduling regular check-ups with your healthcare provider. Blood tests provide objective data on how peptides are impacting your health.

Hormone Levels: If using growth hormone-stimulating peptides, monitor hormone levels to ensure they remain within a healthy range.

Immune Markers: For immune-focused protocols, check markers like white blood cell count to assess immune resilience.

Metabolic Markers: Track blood glucose, cholesterol, and other metabolic indicators for protocols aimed at longevity and metabolic health.

5. Assess Progress Over Time

Peptides typically work over an extended period, so it's helpful to evaluate your results monthly or quarterly. Consider asking yourself the following:

- Are My Goals Being Met? Evaluate whether you're seeing the results you initially aimed for, whether that's improved skin texture, faster recovery, or increased vitality.
- Do I Need Adjustments? If you're not achieving your desired results, consult your healthcare provider about adjusting dosages or adding complementary peptides.
- Is My Protocol Sustainable? Peptide therapy should be sustainable and integrate smoothly into your life. If the routine feels overwhelming, explore ways to simplify or modify it.

Tips for Making Adjustments

If your progress stalls or you're not seeing the expected benefits, making small adjustments can optimize your peptide regimen.

Change Dosages Gradually:** Increase or decrease doses in small increments rather than making drastic changes. This approach allows you to observe the effects of each adjustment.

Re-Evaluate Protocols Periodically: Every few months, review your goals and current protocol to determine if any changes are needed based on progress.

Consult Your Provider for Advanced Adjustments: Especially with advanced programs, professional guidance can help you fine-tune your regimen and ensure you're receiving optimal benefits.

Following a structured protocol and tracking your progress are essential for getting the most from peptide therapy. By observing changes, recording your results, and adjusting your regimen as needed, you can make informed decisions that keep you on the path toward your health and anti-aging goals.

Chapter 4: Enhancing Peptide Therapy with Lifestyle Habits

4.1 Nutrition to Complement Peptide Therapy

Peptide therapy offers substantial benefits for anti-aging, wellness, and physical vitality, but its effectiveness can be significantly enhanced with the right nutrition. Peptides work on a cellular level, supporting processes like collagen synthesis, tissue repair, immune function, and hormonal balance. Nutrition is a critical factor that fuels these processes and supplies essential nutrients for optimal results. When combined, peptide therapy and a nutrient-rich diet can create a synergistic effect, enhancing both short- and long-term health outcomes.

The Importance of Nutrition in Peptide Therapy

Nutrition is the foundation of health, providing the building blocks necessary for cellular repair, energy production, immune function, and more. Peptides, in turn, support these functions by signaling the body to optimize growth, repair, and rejuvenation. When your body receives the right nutrients, it can respond to peptides more effectively, making the benefits more profound and long-lasting.

Key areas where nutrition complements peptide therapy include:

Supporting Collagen Production: Peptides like GHK-Cu rely on collagen synthesis for skin health, elasticity, and wound healing.

Enhancing Muscle Repair and Growth: Growth hormone-stimulating peptides work alongside amino acids and protein to promote muscle development and recovery.

Optimizing Metabolism: Nutrients that support mitochondrial function, such as B vitamins and antioxidants, work well with metabolic peptides like MOTS-c to boost energy levels and metabolic health.

Balancing Hormones: Healthy fats, vitamins, and minerals play a role in hormonal regulation, supporting peptides that influence hormonal health.

Nutrients to Focus On

Here are some of the most important nutrients that complement peptide therapy, along with food sources that provide them:

1. Protein and Amino Acids

Proteins are essential for repairing tissues, building muscle, and maintaining healthy skin. Peptides that target muscle growth, like CJC-1295 and Ipamorelin, benefit from a high-protein diet that provides essential amino acids.

Key Sources: Lean meats (chicken, turkey, beef), fish (salmon, tuna), eggs, Greek yogurt, and plant-based proteins (lentils, chickpeas, quinoa).
Tips: Aim for a balanced intake of protein throughout the day, including a protein source with each meal to support continuous muscle repair and growth.

2. Antioxidants

Antioxidants reduce oxidative stress, which damages cells and accelerates aging. Peptides like GHK-Cu benefit from antioxidants because they reduce inflammation and protect skin cells.

Key Sources: Berries (blueberries, strawberries), leafy greens (spinach, kale), nuts (almonds, walnuts), and green tea.

Tips: Include a variety of antioxidant-rich foods to provide different types of antioxidants, such as vitamin C, vitamin E, and polyphenols, for comprehensive cellular protection.

3. Healthy Fats

Healthy fats are critical for hormone production, brain health, and cell membrane integrity. Peptides that influence growth hormone and metabolic function work best with a diet that includes omega-3 and monounsaturated fats.

Key Sources: Fatty fish (salmon, sardines), olive oil, avocados, chia seeds, and flaxseeds.
Tips: Incorporate healthy fats in moderation, as they're calorie-dense. A balanced intake of omega-3s and monounsaturated fats can enhance cognitive function, energy, and hormonal health.

4. Vitamins and Minerals

Essential vitamins and minerals support nearly every bodily function, from immune response and skin health to energy production and bone strength. For example, vitamin C and zinc aid collagen production, while magnesium and potassium are vital for muscle function.

Key Sources: Citrus fruits, leafy greens, nuts, seeds, and whole grains.
Tips: A diverse diet rich in fruits and vegetables can help you get a wide array of vitamins and minerals that support peptide function.

5. Hydration

Hydration is often overlooked but is essential for nutrient transport, cell health, and energy production. Peptides that enhance metabolic function, muscle recovery, and skin elasticity require adequate hydration to work effectively.

Tips: Aim for 8-10 glasses of water per day, adjusting based on your activity level and climate. Consider hydrating foods like watermelon, cucumber, and celery as part of your fluid intake.

Structuring a Diet to Enhance Peptide Therapy

Designing a meal plan that aligns with your peptide therapy goals doesn't need to be complicated. Here's a sample structure for meals that support peptide function, tailored to various goals.

Sample Meal Plan: Supporting Muscle Growth and Recovery

Breakfast: Greek yogurt with berries, chia seeds, and a handful of almonds for protein and antioxidants.
Lunch: Grilled chicken salad with mixed greens, quinoa, avocado, and a drizzle of olive oil.
Snack: Protein smoothie with spinach, a banana, protein powder, and a scoop of flaxseeds.
Dinner: Salmon with steamed broccoli, sweet potato, and a side of mixed vegetables for balanced macronutrients.

Sample Meal Plan: Boosting Skin Health and Anti-Aging

Breakfast: Smoothie with blueberries, spinach, Greek yogurt, and a teaspoon of honey for natural antioxidants and collagen-boosting nutrients.
Lunch: Avocado and mixed vegetable salad with lean turkey, drizzled with extra virgin olive oil for healthy fats.
Snack: A handful of walnuts and an apple for omega-3s and hydration.
Dinner: Grilled fish with a side of asparagus, quinoa, and a mixed greens salad.

Supplements to Complement Peptide Therapy

While whole foods are the best source of nutrients, certain supplements can complement peptide therapy, especially if you have specific health needs.

Collagen Powder: Supports skin health, joint function, and elasticity.
Vitamin D and K2: Helps maintain bone health and supports immune function.
Omega-3 Fatty Acids: Essential for brain health, reducing inflammation, and supporting heart health.
Magnesium: Aids muscle function, reduces inflammation, and promotes relaxation.

Key Takeaways for Nutrition and Peptide Therapy

1. Prioritize Whole Foods: Opt for nutrient-dense, whole foods that offer a range of vitamins, minerals, and antioxidants to complement peptides.

2. Include Protein at Every Meal: Protein supports muscle recovery and collagen production, making it essential for peptide regimens focused on muscle growth or anti-aging.

3. Balance Macronutrients: Aim for a balanced intake of protein, healthy fats, and carbohydrates to fuel energy, cell repair, and metabolic health.

4. Stay Consistent: Regularly consuming nutrient-rich foods will support peptide therapy's long-term effects, helping you achieve your health and anti-aging goals.

By following these nutritional principles, you can create a diet that supports your peptide therapy regimen, enhancing the results of your efforts and providing a foundation for sustained wellness and vitality.

4.2 Exercise Regimens to Boost Youthful Vitality

Exercise is one of the most powerful tools for enhancing physical vitality and promoting longevity, and it's an excellent companion to peptide therapy. Just as peptides support muscle growth, fat metabolism, and cellular repair, exercise activates these same processes, creating a reinforcing loop that amplifies the benefits of both. Regular exercise improves cardiovascular health, strengthens muscles, boosts energy, and sharpens mental focus—all of which contribute to a youthful appearance and enhanced resilience against aging.

The Role of Exercise in Anti-Aging and Peptide Therapy

Exercise has unique effects on the body that go beyond simple calorie burning. It helps preserve lean muscle mass, stimulates the release of growth hormone, improves blood circulation, and reduces oxidative stress—all of which are vital for combating the effects of aging. When combined with peptides that support growth hormone release, muscle repair, and metabolism, exercise becomes a powerful driver of anti-aging and wellness.

Key benefits of exercise in the context of peptide therapy include:

Enhanced Growth Hormone Production: Exercise, especially resistance training and high-intensity interval training (HIIT), naturally boosts growth hormone levels. This complements peptides like CJC-1295 and Ipamorelin, which are designed to increase growth hormone, supporting muscle growth and recovery.

Improved Circulation and Nutrient Delivery: Physical activity enhances blood flow, delivering oxygen and nutrients to muscles, skin, and organs. Peptides like GHK-Cu benefit from improved circulation as it supports collagen synthesis and skin rejuvenation.

Increased Mitochondrial Function and Metabolism: Exercise stimulates mitochondria, the energy powerhouses of cells, helping to support metabolic peptides like MOTS-c that enhance cellular energy production.

Stress Reduction and Mental Clarity: Exercise releases endorphins, which reduce stress and improve mood, supporting the holistic effects of peptides aimed at cognitive and mental health.

Types of Exercise to Support Youthful Vitality

To maximize the benefits of peptide therapy, incorporating a variety of exercise types is essential. Different types of exercise stimulate different physiological processes, creating a balanced program that supports muscle tone, endurance, flexibility, and mental well-being.

1. Strength Training

Strength training is key for building and preserving lean muscle, improving bone density, and increasing metabolic rate. As we age, maintaining muscle mass becomes critical for strength, stability, and metabolic health. Peptides that stimulate growth hormone release, such as CJC-1295 and Ipamorelin, work particularly well when paired with strength training.

Recommended Frequency: 2-4 times per week, depending on experience level.

Exercises: Focus on compound movements that target multiple muscle groups, such as squats, deadlifts, lunges, bench presses, and rows. These exercises promote muscle hypertrophy and overall strength.

Tips: Start with a weight that challenges you but allows for proper form. Gradually increase weight or reps as you build strength to continually stimulate muscle growth and metabolism.

2. High-Intensity Interval Training (HIIT)

HIIT is a time-efficient exercise method that alternates between short bursts of intense activity and brief rest periods. This type of training boosts cardiovascular health, burns fat, and increases growth hormone production, making it a valuable addition to a peptide regimen focused on metabolic health.

Recommended Frequency: 1-2 times per week.
Exercises: Include exercises like sprints, jumping jacks, kettlebell swings, or cycling sprints. Aim for 20-30 seconds of intense effort followed by 10-20 seconds of rest, repeating for 15-20 minutes.
Tips: HIIT can be demanding, so listen to your body and adjust the intensity as needed. This approach maximizes calorie burn in a short period, supporting both fat loss and cardiovascular health.

3. Cardiovascular Exercise

Cardio exercises like brisk walking, cycling, and swimming support heart health, improve circulation, and enhance endurance. While less intense than strength training or HIIT, cardio is essential for maintaining a balanced fitness routine and complements peptides that support cardiovascular and metabolic health.

Recommended Frequency: 3-5 times per week, with at least one moderate-to-high-intensity session.

Exercises: Walking, jogging, cycling, and swimming are excellent options. Try to incorporate one longer session (30-45 minutes) per week for endurance.

Tips: Vary your cardio activities to prevent boredom and avoid overuse injuries. Low-impact options like swimming or cycling are gentler on joints and can be particularly beneficial for longevity.

4. Flexibility and Mobility Exercises

Flexibility exercises enhance joint mobility, reduce stiffness, and improve overall movement quality. Stretching and mobility work support muscle recovery and reduce the risk of injury, which is essential for sustaining an active lifestyle. Peptides like BPC-157, known for healing and reducing inflammation, work well alongside flexibility exercises.

Recommended Frequency: 2-3 times per week or daily if possible.

Exercises: Yoga, dynamic stretching, and foam rolling are effective options. Focus on stretching major muscle groups such as hamstrings, hip flexors, shoulders, and back.

Tips: Warm up with dynamic stretches before workouts and cool down with static stretches after. This approach prepares muscles for exercise and supports post-workout recovery.

Sample Exercise Regimens to Complement Peptide Therapy

Here are sample weekly routines tailored for different fitness levels. These regimens incorporate a balance of strength, cardio, and flexibility training, alignàing well with the benefits of peptide therapy.

Beginner Routine

- **Monday:** Light cardio (30-minute brisk walk or cycle).
- **Wednesday:** Full-body strength training (squats, push-ups, rows).
- **Friday:** HIIT session (10-15 minutes, low intensity).
- **Saturday:** Flexibility work (15-minute stretch or yoga).

This routine introduces strength, cardio, and flexibility at a moderate intensity, allowing new exercisers to build consistency while supporting peptides focused on muscle growth and recovery.

Intermediate Routine

- **Monday:** Strength training (upper body focus—bench press, rows, shoulder press).
- **Tuesday:** 30-minute moderate cardio (jogging or cycling).
- **Thursday:** Strength training (lower body focus—squats, lunges, deadlifts).

- **Friday:** HIIT session (20 minutes, moderate intensity).
- **Saturday:** Flexibility work (dynamic stretching and foam rolling).

This routine builds on the beginner program by increasing intensity and adding variety. It complements growth hormone-stimulating peptides and supports improved muscle tone, metabolism, and recovery.

Advanced Routine

- **Monday:** Strength training (push focus—bench press, shoulder press, triceps).
- **Tuesday:** HIIT session (30 minutes, high intensity).
- **Wednesday:** Strength training (pull focus—pull-ups, rows, bicep curls).
- **Thursday:** Cardio endurance (45-minute run or cycle).
- **Friday:** Strength training (lower body—squats, deadlifts, lunges).
- **Saturday:** Flexibility and mobility work (yoga or Pilates, 30 minutes).

This regimen challenges all aspects of fitness—strength, endurance, and flexibility—while supporting the muscle repair and anti-inflammatory benefits of peptides. Advanced users can adjust workout intensity to ensure consistent progress.

Tips for Optimizing Exercise Results with Peptide Therapy

1. Listen to Your Body: Exercise is beneficial, but overtraining can lead to burnout and injury. Balance intense workouts with rest days and low-intensity activities to allow muscles to recover fully.

2. Stay Consistent: Peptide benefits, like exercise gains, develop over time. Commit to your routine consistently, allowing both peptides and exercise to work in harmony for long-term results.

3. Hydrate and Fuel Properly: Proper hydration and a balanced diet are essential for energy, muscle recovery, and effective exercise performance. Aim for a mix of carbohydrates, protein, and healthy fats to fuel your workouts.

4. Focus on Quality Over Quantity: Performing exercises with proper form is more effective and safer than pushing through a high volume of reps with poor technique. Prioritize good form, particularly with weight training.

5. Use Recovery Tools: Foam rolling, massage, and stretching can speed up recovery, reduce soreness, and improve flexibility, complementing peptides like BPC-157 that support joint and muscle health.

Tracking Your Progress and Adjusting as Needed

Exercise benefits are most noticeable over time, so tracking your progress can be motivating and help you identify areas to improve.

Monitor Strength Gains: Record weights, reps, and sets to track strength increases over time.

Track Cardiovascular Endurance: Use a fitness app to measure distances, speeds, and heart rate for cardio sessions.

Assess Flexibility: Note your progress in range of motion or ease of movement in stretches and mobility exercises.

If you're seeing steady progress, continue with your current regimen. If results plateau or you experience discomfort, consult a fitness professional or adjust the intensity and variety of your exercises.

Combining peptide therapy with a balanced exercise regimen creates a powerful foundation for youthful vitality and resilience. By incorporating strength, cardio, and flexibility into your weekly routine, you'll not only enhance the effects of peptides but also improve energy, muscle tone, and overall health. Whether you're just starting or aiming for advanced fitness goals, exercise remains an essential partner in your anti-aging journey, helping you stay active, vibrant, and ready for life's challenges.

4.3 Maximizing Sleep and Recovery for Anti-Aging

Sleep is essential to every aspect of health, impacting cognitive function, mood, immune resilience, and cellular repair. Quality sleep is also one of the most potent anti-aging tools, providing the body and mind with the recovery time needed to repair and rejuvenate. For individuals using peptides as part of an anti-aging or wellness regimen, sleep plays an even more critical role, as peptides designed for muscle recovery, growth hormone release, and immune support are most effective when paired with adequate rest.

Why Sleep is Essential for Anti-Aging and Peptide Therapy

During sleep, the body goes through several stages, including light sleep, deep sleep, and REM (rapid eye movement) sleep. Each stage has unique functions that contribute to physical recovery, mental clarity, and emotional well-being. Peptides like CJC-1295 and Ipamorelin, which stimulate growth hormone release, are most effective during deep sleep, when growth hormone levels peak naturally.

Key benefits of sleep that support anti-aging include:

1. Cellular Repair and Regeneration: During deep sleep, the body releases growth hormone, which aids in tissue repair, muscle growth, and collagen synthesis. These processes are essential for maintaining muscle tone, skin elasticity, and joint health.
2. Immune Function Enhancement: Sleep supports immune health by promoting the production of cytokines, proteins that help combat infections and inflammation. Peptides like Thymosin Beta-4 and BPC-157, which support immune function, work optimally when paired with sufficient sleep.
3. Cognitive and Emotional Health: REM sleep is critical for memory consolidation, mood regulation, and cognitive clarity. Peptides that support mental health, like those that

enhance mitochondrial function, benefit from the brain's ability to rest and recharge during sleep.

4. Metabolic Health and Hormonal Balance: Sleep regulates hunger hormones like leptin and ghrelin, which influence appetite and metabolism. Peptides that support metabolic function, like MOTS-c, work best when sleep patterns are stable, allowing for better energy regulation and fat metabolism.

Strategies for Maximizing Sleep Quality

Improving sleep quality requires more than just clocking in enough hours. By creating an environment and routine that supports deep, restorative sleep, you can enhance both the effects of peptide therapy and your overall health.

1. Establish a Consistent Sleep Schedule

Consistency is one of the most important factors for achieving quality sleep. By going to bed and waking up at the same time each day, you align your body's internal clock, or circadian rhythm, which regulates sleep-wake cycles.

Tip: Aim for 7-9 hours of sleep each night, adjusting based on how rested you feel upon waking. Try to maintain the same schedule even on weekends to keep your circadian rhythm stable.

2. Create a Restful Sleep Environment

Your bedroom environment plays a significant role in sleep quality. Dark, quiet, and cool spaces are ideal for deep sleep, as they limit distractions and promote relaxation.

Temperature: Keep the room between 60-67°F (15-19°C), as cooler temperatures promote deeper sleep.
Lighting: Use blackout curtains to block out light, or wear a sleep mask. Dim the lights an hour before bedtime to signal your body that it's time to wind down.
Noise: Reduce noise with earplugs or a white noise machine if needed. Consistent, low-level sounds can be soothing and help mask disruptive noises.

3. Avoid Stimulants Before Bedtime

Stimulants like caffeine and nicotine can disrupt sleep by increasing alertness and delaying the onset of deep sleep. It's best to limit these substances in the afternoon and evening to support restful sleep.

Tip: Limit caffeine intake to the morning hours, and avoid alcohol at least two hours before bed, as it can interfere with REM sleep and reduce overall sleep quality.

4. Establish a Relaxing Pre-Sleep Routine

Creating a pre-sleep routine signals your body that it's time to relax, helping you transition into sleep more easily. Engaging in calming activities, like reading, meditating, or gentle stretching, can reduce stress and promote a smoother transition to sleep.

Ideas for a Routine: Try activities like deep breathing exercises, journaling, or taking a warm bath to relax both your body and mind.

Limit Screen Time: Avoid screens (phones, computers, TVs) an hour before bed, as blue light suppresses melatonin, a hormone that regulates sleep. If screen use is unavoidable, consider using blue light-blocking glasses.

5. Incorporate Sleep-Supporting Nutrients

Certain nutrients, like magnesium, melatonin, and L-theanine, have been shown to promote relaxation and improve sleep quality. These supplements can be particularly helpful when starting a new sleep routine or dealing with occasional insomnia.

Magnesium: Helps relax muscles and calm the nervous system, promoting better sleep.

Melatonin: A natural sleep hormone that can be useful for regulating sleep cycles, especially for individuals experiencing jet lag or irregular sleep patterns.

L-theanine: An amino acid found in green tea that promotes relaxation without sedation, making it useful for pre-sleep anxiety.

Aligning Peptide Therapy with Sleep for Optimal Results

Many peptides work most effectively when administered at night, as they complement the body's natural nighttime repair processes. Here's how to align specific peptides with sleep routines to maximize their benefits.

Peptides to Take Before Bedtime

1. CJC-1295 and Ipamorelin: These peptides stimulate growth hormone release, which is naturally highest during deep sleep. Administering them 30-60 minutes before bedtime allows them to work in harmony with your body's natural growth hormone peak.

2. Epitalon: Known for its anti-aging effects on cellular health and telomeres, Epitalon is often used at night to support longevity and regeneration.

3. Thymosin Beta-4: For those focused on immune health and recovery, Thymosin Beta-4's regenerative effects are enhanced by restful sleep, making nighttime a good time to administer it.

Tracking Sleep Patterns to Assess Peptide Efficacy

Tracking your sleep patterns can offer insights into how well peptides are working, especially those focused on recovery, immune health, or growth hormone release. Many sleep-tracking apps and wearable devices provide data on sleep stages, allowing you to observe improvements over time.

Key Metrics: Look at sleep duration, sleep efficiency, and time spent in deep and REM sleep stages. Improvement in these areas may indicate better recovery, immune resilience, and overall energy.

Adjust Based on Results: If you notice a decline in sleep quality after starting a peptide, consult a healthcare provider for dosage adjustments or consider shifting peptide timing.

Addressing Common Sleep Disruptions

Despite best efforts, sleep disruptions can occur due to stress, travel, or changes in routine. Here are some strategies for overcoming common sleep obstacles.

1. Managing Stress and Anxiety

Stress and anxiety are leading causes of sleep difficulties. Engaging in stress-reducing practices, like mindfulness meditation, deep breathing, or journaling, can help quiet the mind before bed.

Peptides for Support: Peptides that support cognitive function and mental clarity, like those targeting mitochondrial health, can indirectly improve resilience against stress.

2. Dealing with Jet Lag and Shift Work

Traveling across time zones or working irregular hours can disrupt the body's circadian rhythm. To combat jet lag, consider gradually adjusting your sleep schedule to align with your destination's time zone before you travel.

Melatonin: Taking melatonin supplements can help reset the body's internal clock, making it easier to adjust to a new sleep schedule.

Epitalon: Known for its role in circadian rhythm regulation, Epitalon may offer additional support for adapting to changes in time zones or sleep schedules.

3. Improving Sleep During Menopause

Menopause can impact sleep quality due to hormonal fluctuations. Strategies such as cooling the room, wearing breathable fabrics, and practicing relaxation techniques can help alleviate symptoms like hot flashes and night sweats that interrupt sleep.

Nutritional Support: Foods rich in phytoestrogens, like flaxseeds and soy, may help balance hormones naturally. Peptides that support hormone health may also be beneficial, as they work alongside dietary efforts to stabilize symptoms.

Key Takeaways for Enhancing Sleep with Peptide Therapy

1. Prioritize Consistent, Quality Sleep: Establishing regular sleep patterns maximizes peptide benefits, as restful sleep supports growth hormone release, immune function, and cellular repair.

2. Optimize Pre-Sleep Routines: Creating a relaxing bedtime routine, free from stimulants and stressors, enhances your body's ability to achieve deep, restorative sleep.

3. Track Progress: Monitoring sleep metrics helps you observe how peptides are impacting recovery and energy, providing valuable feedback for refining your regimen.

4. Align Peptide Timing: Administering certain peptides before bed can amplify their effectiveness, especially those focused on growth hormone release, immune support, and cellular health.

By enhancing sleep quality, you can create the ideal conditions for peptide therapy to work its best, allowing you to wake up refreshed, revitalized, and ready to embrace each day with energy and resilience.

4.4 A Holistic Approach: Integrating Mind, Body, and Peptides

Peptide therapy offers a powerful avenue for promoting vitality, resilience, and youthfulness, but its effectiveness can be greatly enhanced through a holistic approach that incorporates mental, emotional, and physical wellness. When the body and mind are in harmony, peptides work synergistically with lifestyle habits to yield more profound and sustainable results. Holistic wellness is about creating a balanced life that integrates physical health, mental clarity, emotional well-being, and meaningful connections, allowing you to experience the full benefits of anti-aging efforts.

The Role of Holistic Wellness in Anti-Aging

Holistic wellness is based on the idea that true health goes beyond just the physical body. The mind, emotions, environment, and even social connections play integral roles in shaping our health and how we age. By incorporating mindful practices, stress management, positive relationships, and a sense of purpose, we can create an environment where peptide therapy works to its fullest potential.

Key components of holistic wellness that support anti-aging include:

1. Mental Clarity and Mindfulness: Practices like meditation, journaling, and mindfulness help manage stress, enhance focus, and improve emotional resilience, creating a balanced mental state that complements physical health.

2. Emotional Balance and Stress Reduction: Emotions have a powerful impact on the body's physiological responses. Reducing chronic stress and enhancing emotional well-being supports immune health, hormone balance, and energy levels, all of which play a role in aging.

3. Social Connections and Support: Meaningful relationships and social support have been shown to improve mental health, reduce stress, and even enhance longevity. Feeling connected and supported contributes to an overall sense of well-being and optimism.

4. Purpose and Fulfillment: Having a sense of purpose positively impacts longevity, motivation, and overall happiness. Engaging in meaningful activities fosters resilience, helps manage life's challenges, and promotes a healthy outlook.

Practices for Integrating Mind, Body, and Peptides

By combining peptide therapy with lifestyle habits that nourish the mind and body, you can create a balanced, comprehensive approach to aging gracefully. Below are some practices that support this integration.

1. Mindfulness and Meditation for Stress Reduction

Mindfulness and meditation are effective tools for reducing stress, enhancing focus, and promoting mental clarity. Chronic stress can accelerate aging by increasing inflammation, disturbing sleep, and affecting hormone balance. Peptides that support cognitive function, immune health, and metabolism benefit from a calm, balanced mental state.

Daily Meditation: Spend 5-10 minutes each morning in meditation, focusing on your breath and bringing awareness to the present moment. Meditation helps to reduce cortisol, a stress hormone that impacts skin, immune health, and metabolism.

Mindful Breathing: Practicing deep, mindful breathing throughout the day helps calm the nervous system. Simple techniques, such as inhaling for four counts, holding for four, and exhaling for six, can quickly reduce stress and increase focus.

2. Positive Relationships and Social Engagement

Building and maintaining positive relationships contributes to a strong support system, which promotes emotional well-being and resilience. Peptides that focus on immune support and mental clarity benefit from a healthy, stress-free environment enriched by supportive relationships.

Stay Connected: Regularly connect with friends and family, whether through calls, social gatherings, or activities you enjoy together. These interactions provide emotional support, reduce feelings of isolation, and enhance overall well-being.

Engage in Group Activities: Join a class, club, or community group that aligns with your interests. Group activities provide a sense of belonging, foster social engagement, and encourage shared experiences that enhance life satisfaction.

3. Purposeful Living and Goal Setting

A strong sense of purpose has been linked to improved health, longevity, and emotional resilience. Pursuing meaningful goals provides motivation, reduces stress, and enhances mental clarity, creating an ideal environment for peptides focused on anti-aging and mental wellness.

Set Long-Term Goals: Identify what brings you joy and fulfillment, whether it's learning a new skill, engaging in a hobby, or contributing to your community. Working toward meaningful goals creates a sense of direction, which contributes to emotional and mental health.

Practice Gratitude: Taking time each day to reflect on what you're grateful for has been shown to improve mood, reduce stress, and enhance overall happiness. Try keeping a gratitude journal and noting three things you're thankful for each day.

4. Mind-Body Exercise for Physical and Mental Health

Mind-body exercises like yoga, Pilates, and tai chi combine movement with mindful breathing, creating a bridge between physical fitness and mental clarity. These practices promote flexibility, balance, and strength while also reducing stress, all of which support anti-aging efforts and complement peptide therapy.

Yoga: Yoga combines strength and flexibility with mindful breathing and meditation. It helps improve circulation, reduce muscle tension, and promote relaxation, which benefits both the mind and body.

Tai Chi: Often referred to as "meditation in motion," tai chi enhances balance, flexibility, and relaxation. It's particularly beneficial for individuals looking to improve coordination, relieve stress, and promote joint health.

5. Creative Expression for Emotional Release

Engaging in creative activities, such as painting, writing, or music, provides an outlet for emotional expression and stress relief. Creative expression helps process emotions, reduce anxiety, and improve self-awareness, contributing to an overall sense of well-being.

Art and Music: Expressive arts like drawing, painting, or playing an instrument can be therapeutic, reducing stress and improving focus. This form of release is particularly beneficial for emotional resilience, helping individuals handle challenges more effectively.

Writing and Journaling: Journaling allows you to express thoughts and emotions freely, helping to process stress and gain clarity. Regular journaling provides insights into your mental and emotional state, enhancing self-awareness and promoting mental health.

Creating a Holistic Routine That Complements Peptide Therapy

For a truly integrated approach, consider building a daily or weekly routine that includes practices to support physical, mental, and emotional wellness. Here's an example of a well-rounded weekly routine that aligns with peptide therapy goals.

Sample Holistic Weekly Routine

- **Daily:**

Morning: 5-10 minutes of meditation, followed by a balanced breakfast rich in protein and healthy fats.

Midday: Take time for a mindful walk or short stretching session to reset and reduce stress.

Evening: Engage in a relaxation activity, like reading or gentle yoga, before bedtime. Administer bedtime peptides (like CJC-1295 or Ipamorelin) as recommended.

- **Weekly:**

Strength and Cardio Workouts: 3-4 days of strength training and cardiovascular exercise to maintain muscle tone, improve metabolism, and boost energy.

Social Engagement: Schedule time to connect with friends or family, whether for a meal, outdoor activity, or simply a chat.

Creative Expression or Learning: Dedicate time to a creative activity or skill-building that brings you joy and satisfaction.

Mind-Body Exercise: Practice yoga, tai chi, or stretching 1-2 times per week to enhance flexibility, focus, and relaxation.

Peptides That Align with a Holistic Lifestyle

Certain peptides work especially well when combined with holistic lifestyle practices, as they support mental clarity, cellular health, and emotional resilience.

1. Epitalon: Known for its effects on longevity and circadian rhythm regulation, Epitalon works synergistically with practices that support sleep, reduce stress, and promote cellular health.
2. GHK-Cu: A peptide known for skin and tissue repair, GHK-Cu supports a balanced lifestyle that includes antioxidant-rich nutrition and relaxation practices that reduce oxidative stress.
3. BPC-157: With its anti-inflammatory properties, BPC-157 complements a routine focused on mind-body balance, supporting joint health, recovery, and overall physical resilience.

Key Takeaways for a Holistic Anti-Aging Approach

1. Integrate Mindful Practices: Combining meditation, creative expression, and mental clarity exercises with peptide therapy enhances overall well-being, creating a balanced mental state.
2. Cultivate Positive Relationships: Engaging in supportive relationships promotes mental health and resilience, reducing stress and fostering optimism.
3. Pursue a Sense of Purpose: Meaningful goals and daily gratitude create motivation and emotional resilience, essential components of a fulfilling life.

4. Engage in Mind-Body Activities: Practices like yoga, tai chi, and gentle stretching connect the mind and body, improving flexibility, reducing tension, and supporting peptides focused on physical health.

By incorporating a holistic approach to wellness, you create the ideal conditions for peptide therapy to work synergistically with the mind, body, and spirit. This integration not only enhances physical health but also fosters a deep sense of well-being, helping you age gracefully, stay resilient, and live life with a sense of purpose and joy.

Chapter 5: The Mental Side of Aging – Mindfulness and Motivation

5.1 Stress Management and Its Role in Aging

Aging isn't solely a physical process; it's profoundly influenced by mental and emotional health. One of the most impactful aspects of mental wellness is how we manage stress. Chronic stress can accelerate aging on a cellular level, leading to inflammation, hormonal imbalances, reduced immune function, and even visible signs of aging like wrinkles and fatigue. Managing stress effectively is, therefore, a critical component of any anti-aging strategy, working alongside peptide therapy and healthy lifestyle habits to promote long-term resilience and vitality.

How Stress Affects the Aging Process

Stress triggers a cascade of physiological responses designed to protect the body in short-term, high-stress situations. However, when stress becomes chronic, these responses continue unchecked, leading to wear and tear on the body over time. Chronic stress is linked to a range of negative effects that accelerate aging, affecting everything from the immune system to skin health.

Key areas where stress impacts aging include:

1. Hormonal Imbalance: Stress triggers the release of cortisol, a hormone that regulates our *"fight-or-flight"* response. While cortisol is essential in small amounts, chronic elevations can disrupt hormonal balance, leading to inflammation, blood sugar imbalances, and even loss of muscle tone.
2. Cellular Aging and Telomere Shortening: Chronic stress has been shown to shorten telomeres, the protective caps at the ends of chromosomes. Telomere shortening accelerates cellular aging, increasing the risk of age-related diseases and reducing lifespan.
3. Immune Function Suppression: High stress levels suppress immune function, making the body more vulnerable to infections and reducing its ability to repair and regenerate. This impacts everything from muscle recovery to skin health.
4. Increased Oxidative Stress: Stress increases oxidative stress, which damages cells, proteins, and DNA. This oxidative damage is a major contributor to the aging process,

impacting skin elasticity, energy levels, and cognitive function.

Practical Strategies for Managing Stress to Support Anti-Aging

Managing stress is essential for preserving youthful vitality and maximizing the benefits of peptide therapy. Here are some effective techniques to help reduce stress and create a balanced mental state that supports healthy aging.

1. Practice Deep Breathing Exercises: Deep breathing exercises activate the body's relaxation response, lowering cortisol levels and promoting a state of calm. These exercises can be done anywhere and take only a few minutes, making them an accessible tool for managing stress.

How to Practice: Try the 4-7-8 breathing technique: inhale through your nose for a count of four, hold the breath for a count of seven, and exhale through your mouth for a count of eight. Repeat 3-5 times.
Benefits: Deep breathing improves oxygen delivery to cells, reduces heart rate, and triggers the body's natural relaxation response.

2. Engage in Physical Activity: Exercise is one of the most effective ways to reduce stress and improve mood, thanks to the release of endorphins—natural mood-boosting chemicals. Regular physical activity also supports peptide therapy by promoting muscle health, increasing circulation, and enhancing metabolic function.

Recommended Activities: Walking, jogging, yoga, and strength training are all excellent options. Aim for at least 150 minutes of moderate exercise per week.

Tips: Choose activities you enjoy to make exercise a positive part of your daily routine, reducing stress while promoting physical health.

3. Establish Healthy Boundaries: Modern life often brings a constant stream of demands, from work obligations to social responsibilities. Learning to set healthy boundaries—knowing when to say "no"—helps prevent burnout and reduces chronic stress.

How to Set Boundaries: Prioritize tasks based on importance and align your commitments with your values. Communicate your needs assertively, ensuring you have time for self-care and rest.

Benefits: Healthy boundaries reduce overwhelm, promote work-life balance, and create mental space for relaxation and rejuvenation.

4. Use Relaxation Techniques for Daily Stress Relief: Incorporating relaxation techniques like progressive muscle relaxation (PMR), visualization, and guided imagery into your routine helps release tension and calm the mind.

Progressive Muscle Relaxation: Focus on tensing and relaxing each muscle group, working from the toes to the head. This practice reduces physical tension and brings awareness to areas of the body that may be holding stress.

Visualization and Imagery: Imagine yourself in a peaceful, calming place, engaging all your senses to deepen relaxation. Guided imagery apps can help facilitate this process.

5. Limit Exposure to Stress Triggers: Identify and minimize exposure to stress triggers, particularly if they are avoidable or can be managed. This might include limiting news consumption, managing social media use, or practicing mindfulness in situations that typically cause stress.

Benefits: Reducing exposure to triggers helps control cortisol levels, contributing to overall mental clarity and calm.
Tip: Practice mindfulness techniques, focusing on the present moment, to reduce reactivity to stressful situations.

Key Takeaways for Effective Stress Management

1. Adopt Mindfulness Practices: Techniques like deep breathing and meditation help reduce cortisol, promoting a calm mental state that supports anti-aging efforts.
2. Maintain a Balanced Lifestyle: Exercise, healthy boundaries, and self-care reduce stress, supporting mental clarity and resilience.
3. Use Relaxation Techniques Regularly: Consistent use of relaxation techniques helps build resilience to stress, keeping the body's stress response under control.

By adopting stress management practices, you create an internal environment that supports the benefits of peptide therapy, helping you age gracefully with resilience, energy, and peace of mind.

5.2 Mindfulness Techniques to Enhance Anti-Aging Efforts

Mindfulness, the practice of being fully present and engaged in the moment, has gained widespread attention for its profound effects on mental and physical health. Mindfulness practices reduce stress, improve emotional resilience, and enhance cognitive function, all of which contribute to a more youthful, resilient state of being. In the context of anti-aging, mindfulness provides tools to slow down mental aging, support emotional balance, and promote mental clarity, aligning well with the goals of peptide therapy and a healthy lifestyle.

The Connection Between Mindfulness and Anti-Aging

Mindfulness is more than a mental exercise—it has direct physiological benefits that support anti-aging. Regular mindfulness practice has been shown to improve sleep, reduce inflammation, and enhance immune function, all of which are vital for slowing the aging process. Mindfulness positively affects areas such as:

1. Cognitive Function: Mindfulness promotes mental clarity, memory, and focus, helping protect against cognitive decline as we age.

2. Emotional Regulation: Practicing mindfulness enhances emotional resilience, reducing the impact of stress on the body and mind.

3. Physical Health: Mindfulness lowers levels of cortisol and other stress hormones, reducing inflammation and supporting skin, immune, and cardiovascular health.

4. Telomere Preservation: Research has shown that mindfulness can even help preserve telomere length, protecting chromosomes from age-related degradation at the cellular level.

Effective Mindfulness Techniques for Anti-Aging

The following mindfulness techniques are tailored to support a balanced mind and body, enhancing the effects of peptide therapy and creating a foundation for long-term wellness. Each practice can be easily integrated into daily life, helping to cultivate a calm, youthful, and resilient mindset.

1. Breath Awareness Meditation: Breath awareness meditation is a simple yet powerful technique that helps calm the mind, reduce stress, and promote a state of mental clarity. This practice involves focusing on each breath, which activates the parasympathetic nervous system and reduces cortisol levels, fostering a sense of calm and relaxation.

How to Practice: Sit comfortably, close your eyes, and bring your attention to your breath. Inhale deeply through your nose, noticing the sensation of air entering your lungs, then exhale slowly. Continue for 5-10 minutes, gently refocusing on your breath if your mind wanders.

Benefits: Regular breath awareness helps build resilience to stress, reduces blood pressure, and supports cognitive clarity.

2. Body Scan Meditation: Body scan meditation involves mentally scanning each part of your body, noticing sensations without judgment. This practice fosters body awareness, relieves physical tension, and promotes relaxation. The technique can be particularly beneficial for supporting peptide therapy focused on muscle recovery and inflammation reduction.

How to Practice: Lie down comfortably and close your eyes. Begin at the top of your head and mentally scan down through each body part, from head to toe, paying attention to any sensations or areas of tension. Spend a few moments on each area, consciously releasing tension before moving on.
Benefits: Body scan meditation enhances relaxation, reduces muscle tension, and improves sleep quality.

3. Mindful Walking: Mindful walking combines movement with mindfulness, helping reduce mental clutter and promoting a deeper connection with your environment. This practice can be especially grounding, reducing anxiety and improving mood, both of which contribute to a positive mindset and emotional resilience.

How to Practice: Find a quiet space and walk at a comfortable pace, focusing on the sensation of each step. Notice how your feet connect with the ground and the rhythm of your movements. Engage your senses by paying attention to sounds, smells, or sights around you.

Benefits: Mindful walking enhances physical and mental relaxation, promoting cardiovascular health and providing a break from the demands of daily life.

4. Loving-Kindness Meditation: Loving-kindness meditation **(also called "metta" meditation)** is a practice of directing positive thoughts and intentions toward yourself and others. This form of meditation fosters empathy, compassion, and a sense of connection, which can enhance emotional resilience and reduce stress-related aging.

How to Practice: Sit quietly and focus on feelings of kindness and compassion. Silently repeat phrases like, ***"May I be happy, may I be healthy, may I live with ease."*** Gradually extend these thoughts to others—loved ones, friends, even strangers.
Benefits: This practice increases emotional resilience, reduces stress, and fosters a sense of positivity and emotional well-being.

5. Visualization and Guided Imagery: Visualization is a technique that involves mentally creating positive, calming images or scenarios. Guided imagery, in particular, can be a powerful tool for relaxation and mental rejuvenation, supporting a youthful, optimistic mindset.

How to Practice: Close your eyes and imagine yourself in a peaceful, serene setting, such as a beach, forest, or mountain. Engage all your senses, imagining the sounds, smells, and sensations of this environment. You can use guided imagery apps or recordings if you're new to visualization.

Benefits: Visualization reduces stress, promotes mental clarity, and provides a mental escape that fosters emotional balance.

Integrating Mindfulness Techniques into Your Daily Routine

For mindfulness to be most effective, consistency is key. Here are some tips for incorporating these techniques into a busy life, so they become natural habits that support mental and physical health.

Create a Morning Mindfulness Routine
Starting your day with mindfulness sets a positive tone and helps you face challenges with resilience. Begin each morning with a 5-10 minute meditation session, whether it's breath awareness, body scan, or visualization, to cultivate a calm and focused mindset.

Tip: Use a meditation app to guide you through a short practice and help you stay consistent.

Practice "Micro-Mindfulness" Moments
Incorporate brief moments of mindfulness throughout your day by practicing mindful breathing, observing your surroundings, or taking a mindful walk. These mini-breaks provide an opportunity to reset, reducing stress and promoting mental clarity.

Example: Take a few deep breaths before a meeting, or focus on the sounds around you while waiting in line. These small moments of awareness contribute to reduced stress and greater emotional balance.

End the Day with a Wind-Down Practice
A bedtime mindfulness routine can improve sleep quality, helping you wind down and release any stress accumulated throughout the day. Practices like loving-kindness meditation or guided imagery are particularly effective for promoting relaxation and a sense of calm before bed.

Tips: Try listening to a guided meditation or soft music as part of your pre-sleep routine, supporting restful, rejuvenating sleep.

Key Takeaways for Mindfulness and Anti-Aging

1. Be Consistent: Regular mindfulness practice helps build emotional resilience, reduce stress, and promote mental clarity, supporting a youthful mindset and physical vitality.
2. Experiment with Different Techniques: Each mindfulness practice offers unique benefits, so try various techniques to see which ones work best for you.
3. Integrate Mindfulness into Daily Life: Making mindfulness a part of daily routines creates a sustainable practice that can be easily maintained, yielding long-term mental and physical benefits.

By incorporating mindfulness practices, you create a balanced mental state that complements peptide therapy, nutrition, and physical wellness, building a comprehensive approach to aging gracefully and vibrantly.

5.3 Setting Anti-Aging Goals and Tracking Success

Setting clear, achievable goals is an essential step in any wellness journey, especially in anti-aging. Goals provide direction, motivation, and a way to measure success over time, ensuring that efforts are focused and progress is visible. For those using peptide therapy, nutrition, exercise, and mindfulness as part of an anti-aging regimen, goal-setting offers a structured approach to monitor improvements and adjust routines as needed. Tracking success keeps you engaged and allows for tangible results, reinforcing the benefits of your anti-aging efforts.

Why Set Anti-Aging Goals?

Anti-aging goals serve as a roadmap to guide your efforts in areas like physical health, mental clarity, and emotional well-being. By setting goals, you create a vision of what you hope to achieve, whether it's improved skin texture, enhanced energy, or greater mental clarity. Goals not only enhance motivation but also allow for self-assessment, helping you adjust and optimize your efforts.

Benefits of goal-setting in anti-aging include:

1. Clarity and Focus: Setting specific goals clarifies your priorities, helping you focus on the areas most important to you.
2. Motivation and Engagement: Goals create a sense of purpose, making it easier to stay consistent with your routine.
3. Measurable Progress: Tracking goals allows you to see the impact of your efforts over time, reinforcing positive changes and revealing areas for improvement.

Steps to Setting Effective Anti-Aging Goals

Effective goal-setting involves creating clear, realistic, and meaningful goals that align with your overall vision for aging gracefully. By following these steps, you can set goals that are motivating, achievable, and tailored to your personal wellness journey.

1. Identify Your Priorities: Start by identifying what aspects of anti-aging are most important to you. This could include physical appearance (e.g., skin health), energy levels, mental clarity, or emotional well-being. Reflect on why each priority matters to you and what improvements would make a positive impact on your life.

Example Goals:
  - Improve skin elasticity and reduce fine lines.
  - Increase muscle tone and physical endurance.
  - Enhance mental clarity and reduce stress levels.

2. Use SMART Goals: SMART goals—Specific, Measurable, Achievable, Relevant, and Time-bound—provide a structured approach to goal-setting that ensures clarity and accountability.

Specific: Define exactly what you want to achieve. Instead of a vague goal like "look younger," specify "reduce visible fine lines on the forehead."

Measurable: Establish how you will track progress, such as tracking skin hydration, muscle mass, or energy levels.

Achievable: Set goals that are challenging but realistic, considering your starting point and available resources.

Relevant: Make sure each goal aligns with your personal priorities and desired anti-aging outcomes.

Time-bound: Give yourself a reasonable timeframe to achieve each goal, like "increase muscle tone within three months."

3. Break Down Goals into Actionable Steps: Large goals can feel overwhelming, so breaking them down into smaller, actionable steps helps maintain momentum and makes each goal more attainable.

Example Breakdown for Improving Skin Health:

   Daily: Apply a peptide serum in the morning and evening, followed by moisturizer.

   Weekly: Incorporate a gentle exfoliating scrub to promote skin cell turnover.

   Monthly: Take "before" and "after" photos to track improvements in skin texture.

4. Set Short-Term and Long-Term Goals: Short-term goals provide quick wins and build momentum, while long-term goals offer a bigger vision for sustained anti-aging progress. Both types of goals play essential roles in creating a balanced approach.

Short-Term Goal: Increase daily water intake to improve skin hydration over the next two weeks.
Long-Term Goal: Improve sleep quality and achieve consistent 8-hour nights within six months, enhancing skin health, mood, and energy.

Tracking Your Anti-Aging Progress

Tracking progress is crucial for assessing the effectiveness of your efforts, providing tangible proof of improvement, and motivating you to continue. Tracking methods can be as simple or detailed as you prefer, but consistency is key for gaining accurate insights.

1. Health and Wellness Journals: A journal dedicated to your anti-aging journey allows you to record daily actions, reflections, and physical changes over time. This can include entries on nutrition, exercise, skincare routines, sleep, and mindfulness practices.

What to Include: Date, specific actions (like skincare application or exercise), observations (e.g., skin tone, mood, energy levels), and reflections on how you feel.

Benefits: Journaling provides a comprehensive record, helping you spot patterns and assess the effects of your anti-aging routine on both mind and body.

2. Progress Photos: Progress photos are an effective way to track physical changes, especially for skin texture, muscle tone, and overall appearance. These images provide a visual record of improvements and help you objectively assess progress.

Tips for Consistency: Take photos at the same time of day, in similar lighting, and from the same angles. For example, take close-ups of your face, upper body, or other areas where you're tracking changes.
Frequency: Consider taking photos every 2-4 weeks to allow enough time for noticeable changes.

 3. Health Tracking Apps and Wearables: Health tracking apps and wearable devices can provide data-driven insights into sleep quality, physical activity, heart rate, and even stress levels. These tools make it easy to monitor progress and adjust goals as needed based on real-time feedback.

Examples of Metrics to Track: Hours of deep sleep, heart rate variability, daily steps, active minutes, and caloric burn.
Benefits: Wearables provide objective data on key health indicators, making it easy to track your progress and make informed adjustments to your routine.

4. Monthly Self-Assessments: Every month, assess your progress by reflecting on each goal and noting areas of improvement or challenges. These self-assessments can help you fine-tune your goals, optimize your routines, and set new objectives as you achieve milestones.

Questions to Consider:
- Have I noticed visible changes in my skin, energy, or mood?
- Am I staying consistent with my daily and weekly routines?
- What adjustments could I make to improve my results?

5. Celebrate Small Wins: Achieving anti-aging goals takes time, and celebrating small successes along the way can help maintain motivation. Whether it's noticing clearer skin or experiencing a surge of energy, acknowledge these moments as markers of progress.

Ideas for Celebrating: Treat yourself to a new skincare product, take a day to relax, or share your achievements with a friend or loved one who supports your journey.

Adjusting Goals as You Progress

As you track progress, you may find that some goals need to be adjusted. Adjusting goals is not a setback—it's a way to stay aligned with your evolving priorities and make the most of what you're learning along the way.

Refine Your Approach: If a particular method isn't yielding the results you hoped for, try experimenting with alternative approaches. For instance, if you're not seeing improvements in skin health with one peptide, consider switching to another.

Increase Challenge Gradually: As you achieve certain goals, raise the bar slightly to keep yourself challenged and motivated. For example, if your goal was to walk 5,000 steps daily, increase it to 7,000 once you're comfortable with the initial goal.

Stay Flexible: Life events, changes in routine, or unexpected challenges can affect progress. Be flexible and adjust timelines or methods as needed, focusing on long-term consistency rather than perfection.

Key Takeaways for Setting Anti-Aging Goals and Tracking Success

1. Set Clear, Realistic Goals: Start by identifying what's most important to you, then break down your goals into achievable, actionable steps.

2. Use Multiple Tracking Methods: Combining journals, progress photos, apps, and self-assessments provides a well-rounded view of your progress.

3. Celebrate Milestones: Acknowledge small wins to maintain motivation and stay engaged with your anti-aging journey.

4. Stay Adaptable: Regularly review and adjust your goals as needed to align with your progress, learning, and lifestyle changes.

By setting intentional goals and tracking your journey, you create a meaningful, motivating framework that makes aging gracefully achievable and rewarding. With each milestone, you'll not only see visible improvements but also feel a greater sense of purpose, fulfillment, and joy in your anti-aging journey.

Chapter 6: Safety First – Minimizing Risks and Managing Side Effects

6.1 Understanding Common Side Effects

As with any wellness intervention, it's essential to prioritize safety when using peptides as part of an anti-aging regimen. While peptides are generally well-tolerated and considered safe for most people, understanding the potential side effects and how to manage them is crucial for a balanced, informed approach to peptide therapy. Knowing what to expect and how to minimize risks enables you to use peptides confidently and effectively, enhancing their benefits while reducing potential downsides.

Why Side Effects Occur in Peptide Therapy

Peptides are short chains of amino acids that naturally occur in the body, making them generally well-tolerated compared to synthetic drugs. However, individual responses to peptides can vary based on factors such as dosage, method of administration, and individual sensitivities. Side effects can arise due to:

1. Immune Response: The body may initially recognize peptides as foreign substances, triggering a mild immune response. This can lead to minor inflammation or irritation.
2. Dosage and Sensitivity: Higher doses increase the risk of side effects, especially in individuals new to peptide therapy or those with sensitive systems.
3. Injection Site Reactions: For peptides administered through injections, mild reactions at the injection site, such as redness or swelling, can occasionally occur.
4. Hormonal Shifts: Peptides that influence hormones, like growth hormone-releasing peptides, may cause temporary hormonal adjustments, leading to mild side effects.

Understanding why side effects happen helps manage expectations and fosters a proactive approach to minimizing risks.

Common Side Effects of Peptide Therapy

Below are some common side effects associated with peptide use, along with strategies to help manage and reduce these effects.

1. Injection Site Reactions:

One of the most frequently reported side effects is mild irritation at the injection site. This can include redness, swelling, tenderness, or itching and usually resolves within a few hours to a day.

Why It Occurs: Injection site reactions occur as the body's natural response to a foreign substance, even though peptides are typically well-accepted. It may also be due to the injection technique or needle size.

How to Manage:
- Use Proper Technique: Follow recommended injection techniques, including disinfecting the area before injection and rotating injection sites to minimize irritation.
- Choose the Right Needle Size: Using a fine-gauge needle (like a 30-31 gauge) can reduce trauma to the skin and minimize discomfort.
- Apply a Cool Compress: After injection, a cool compress can help soothe any mild irritation or swelling.

2. Headaches:
Some peptides, particularly those that stimulate growth hormone release (e.g., CJC-1295 or Ipamorelin), can occasionally cause mild headaches, especially during the initial stages of use.

Why It Occurs: Peptides that influence hormone release can create subtle changes in fluid balance, which may lead to mild headaches in sensitive individuals.

How to Manage:
- Stay Hydrated: Dehydration can exacerbate headaches, so ensure you're drinking plenty of water throughout the day.

- Monitor Dosages: If headaches are frequent, consider lowering the dosage and gradually increasing it as your body adjusts.
- Use Over-the-Counter Pain Relievers: For occasional headaches, standard pain relievers like acetaminophen or ibuprofen can help, but consult with a healthcare provider if headaches persist.

3. Fatigue or Drowsiness:

While many people experience increased energy with peptide therapy, some may feel occasional drowsiness or fatigue, especially with peptides that influence relaxation and growth hormone production.

Why It Occurs: Peptides that boost growth hormone release can influence sleep-wake cycles, potentially leading to mild drowsiness as the body adjusts to increased hormone levels.

How to Manage:
- Time Your Dosage: Administer growth hormone-releasing peptides like CJC-1295 or Ipamorelin before bedtime to align with natural growth hormone peaks during sleep.
- Allow Time for Adjustment: Fatigue often resolves after the body becomes accustomed to peptide use. Monitor energy levels and reduce dosage temporarily if needed.
- Prioritize Rest: If feeling drowsy, consider adjusting your daily activities or incorporating a short nap to manage energy levels.

4. Water Retention:
Water retention, or mild bloating, can occasionally occur, especially with peptides that stimulate growth hormone production. This side effect is generally mild and temporary.

Why It Occurs: Growth hormone has an anabolic effect, which can increase fluid retention in tissues, leading to temporary swelling or puffiness.

How to Manage:
- Monitor Sodium Intake: High sodium intake can exacerbate water retention. Aim to consume balanced meals with low to moderate salt levels.
- Increase Physical Activity: Exercise helps reduce water retention by improving circulation and stimulating lymphatic drainage.
- Reduce Dosage: If water retention is noticeable, consider reducing the peptide dosage and gradually increasing it as your body adjusts.

5. Temporary Mood Changes:
Peptides that influence hormone levels may sometimes affect mood or emotional balance, causing mild shifts like irritability or low mood.

Why It Occurs: Changes in growth hormone, cortisol, and other hormone levels can temporarily impact mood, especially during the body's adjustment period.

How to Manage:
- Engage in Relaxing Activities: Incorporate relaxation practices like meditation, deep breathing, or yoga to support emotional balance.

- Monitor and Adjust Dosage: If mood changes are frequent, consider adjusting the dosage or timing to see if it improves your emotional state.

- Stay Connected: Talking with friends or loved ones can provide support if mood shifts arise, helping you manage emotional responses constructively.

Managing Side Effects: Practical Tips for a Balanced Approach

While most side effects are mild and temporary, a proactive approach can further reduce their likelihood and enhance the overall experience of peptide therapy. Here are some additional strategies for minimizing and managing side effects:

1. Start with a Low Dosage and Gradually Increase:
Starting with a lower dosage allows the body to adjust to peptides gradually, reducing the likelihood of side effects. Once you feel comfortable, you can slowly increase the dosage under the guidance of a healthcare provider.

Tip: If you're new to peptide therapy, begin with the lowest recommended dosage and monitor your response for 1-2 weeks before increasing.

2. Consult with a Healthcare Provider:
A healthcare provider experienced in peptide therapy can help tailor your dosage, suggest timing adjustments, and address any side effects that arise. This personalized guidance reduces the likelihood of adverse reactions and ensures safe usage.

Tip: Schedule regular check-ins with your provider to assess your progress and make any necessary adjustments to your regimen.

3. Monitor Your Body's Response:
Keep track of your experiences in a journal or tracking app. Recording your daily reactions can help you and your healthcare provider identify patterns, understand how your body is responding, and determine whether adjustments are needed.

Tip: Note any side effects, the timing of administration, and other relevant factors, such as diet, sleep, and stress levels, to gain a holistic understanding of your response.

4. Stay Hydrated and Support Your Body with Proper Nutrition:
Staying hydrated and eating a balanced diet can help reduce side effects by supporting metabolic and digestive health. Proper nutrition aids in muscle recovery, hormone regulation, and immune support, creating a stable foundation for peptide therapy.

Tip: Aim for a balanced intake of protein, healthy fats, complex carbohydrates, and plenty of water throughout the day.

5. Practice Good Injection Hygiene and Technique:
For those administering peptides via injection, following proper technique and hygiene is essential to prevent side effects like infections or prolonged irritation.

Tips:
   - Clean the injection area with an alcohol swab before injecting.
   - Rotate injection sites to prevent irritation and ensure even absorption.
   - Dispose of needles safely and avoid reusing needles.

When to Seek Medical Advice

While most side effects are mild, certain symptoms may require consultation with a healthcare provider. It's important to be aware of signs that could indicate a more serious issue, such as:

- Persistent Pain or Swelling: If injection site reactions do not improve or worsen over time, seek advice to rule out infection or allergic response.
- Severe Headaches or Fatigue: Persistent or intense headaches or fatigue that doesn't improve with time should be assessed by a professional.
- Mood or Emotional Changes: If mood shifts become more severe or prolonged, consult your provider to discuss adjustments or additional support.

Key Takeaways for Minimizing Risks and Managing Side Effects

1. Start Low and Go Slow: Gradually increasing dosages helps your body adjust, minimizing the likelihood of side effects.
2. Stay Hydrated and Nourished: Proper hydration and balanced nutrition support your body's response, helping you manage mild side effects.
3. Follow Injection Best Practices: Proper injection technique reduces risks of irritation, infections, and other minor side effects.
4. Track Your Progress: Monitoring your experiences and responses provides valuable feedback for adjusting your regimen as needed.

By understanding common side effects and managing them proactively, you create a safe and effective foundation for peptide therapy. This balanced approach not only enhances your anti-aging journey but also supports your overall well-being, helping you achieve your goals with confidence and clarity.

6.2 Safety Protocols for Peptide Usage

Safety is paramount in any wellness regimen, and peptide therapy is no exception. By following established safety protocols, you can optimize the benefits of peptides while minimizing potential risks. Whether you're new to peptides or have experience with them, adhering to safe practices for dosage, administration, storage, and monitoring is essential for a balanced and effective approach to anti-aging and wellness.

Key Elements of Safe Peptide Usage

The foundation of safe peptide therapy involves paying close attention to four key areas: dosage, administration, storage, and monitoring. Each of these aspects contributes to the efficacy and safety of your regimen, helping you avoid common pitfalls and protect your health.

1. Dosage Management: Taking the correct dosage is essential for achieving desired results while minimizing side effects. Dosages should be based on individual factors like age, weight, health goals, and previous experience with peptides.
2. Proper Administration: Administering peptides correctly, whether by injection, topical application, or oral use, ensures their effectiveness and reduces risks associated with improper technique.
3. Hygiene and Sterility: Hygiene practices are crucial for preventing infections and irritation, especially with injectable peptides. Following sterile practices reduces the risk of complications.
4. Safe Storage: Peptides are sensitive to temperature, light, and contamination, so proper storage is necessary to maintain potency and efficacy over time.

1. Dosage Management

Peptides work best when used at appropriate dosages tailored to individual needs. Starting with a low dose and gradually adjusting it based on your body's response helps achieve a balanced effect while minimizing side effects.

General Dosage Guidelines

- Start Low and Go Slow: Begin with the lowest recommended dosage and increase gradually if needed. This approach allows your body to adjust to peptides, helping to reduce side effects like headaches, fatigue, or mild inflammation.
- Consult with a Healthcare Provider: A healthcare provider can help determine the optimal dosage based on your health status, goals, and experience. They may also recommend periodic blood tests to assess hormone levels and overall wellness.
- Follow Recommended Dosing Intervals: Some peptides are administered daily, while others may be used weekly or in cycles (e.g., 6-8 weeks on, 2-4 weeks off). Adhering to the correct dosing interval helps avoid overstimulation and prevents tolerance buildup.

Dosage Adjustment Protocols

When adjusting dosages, it's essential to track your body's response closely and make gradual changes to avoid sudden reactions.

- Monitor for Side Effects: If you experience mild side effects, consider reducing the dosage and observing any improvements. If side effects persist, consult a healthcare provider.
- Increase Dosages Gradually: For peptides aimed at muscle growth or hormone release, increasing the dosage by small increments (e.g., 10-20%) over a few weeks allows your body to adapt without overwhelming it.
- Adjust Dosages Based on Progress: As you achieve certain goals, such as improved skin elasticity or muscle tone, you may find that you can maintain these results with a lower maintenance dose, reducing the need for higher doses.

2. Proper Administration Techniques

Administering peptides correctly is critical for ensuring they are both safe and effective. The most common methods of administration include injections, topical applications, and oral use, each of which has specific guidelines to follow.

Injectable Peptides: Subcutaneous and Intramuscular

For many peptides, injection is the most effective delivery method because it allows peptides to enter the bloodstream directly, bypassing digestion and ensuring high bioavailability.

- Subcutaneous (Sub-Q) Injections: This method involves injecting peptides into the fatty tissue just under the skin, typically in areas like the abdomen or thigh. Sub-Q injections are less invasive and easier for self-administration.

Technique: Use a fine-gauge needle (e.g., 30-31 gauge) and inject at a 45-degree angle to minimize pain. Clean the injection site with an alcohol swab before and after injection.

Rotation of Injection Sites: Rotate between injection sites to avoid tissue irritation or buildup of scar tissue. For example, alternate between the left and right abdomen.

- Intramuscular (IM) Injections: IM injections are administered directly into muscle tissue, which can result in faster absorption. These injections are typically given in the upper thigh or deltoid (shoulder) muscle.

- **Technique:** Use a slightly larger needle (e.g., 22-25 gauge) and insert it at a 90-degree angle. IM injections are generally better suited for healthcare provider administration, especially for beginners.

- **Consider Professional Guidance:** If you're new to IM injections, consider working with a healthcare provider until you feel comfortable with the process.

Topical Peptides: Application to Skin

Topical peptides are used for localized effects, primarily for skin health, and are applied directly to the skin in the form of creams, serums, or gels.

Application Tips: Cleanse the skin before applying topical peptides to maximize absorption. Gently massage the product into the skin and allow it to absorb fully before applying other skincare products.

Frequency: Most topical peptides can be applied once or twice daily. Follow the product's instructions for best results.

Storage: Some topical peptides may need to be refrigerated to maintain potency, so check storage requirements and avoid exposing the product to heat or sunlight.

Oral Peptides: Capsules and Tablets

Certain peptides are available in oral form, particularly those designed for gut health or metabolic support. While oral peptides may have lower bioavailability due to digestion, they offer a convenient option for users seeking an easy, non-invasive method.

Administration: Take oral peptides as directed, with or without food, depending on the specific peptide's absorption needs.

Tips: Stay consistent with timing (e.g., taking the peptide each morning) to support a stable therapeutic effect.

Consider Bioavailability: Oral peptides may require higher dosages to achieve the same effects as injectable forms. Consult a provider for guidance on dosage.

3. Hygiene and Sterility

For injectable peptides, following proper hygiene protocols is essential to prevent infections, reduce irritation, and ensure safe administration.

Sterility Tips for Injectable Peptides

- Use Fresh, Sterile Needles: Always use a new, sterile needle and syringe for each injection to avoid contamination.

- Disinfect the Injection Site: Clean the injection site with an alcohol swab to remove any bacteria on the skin.
- Avoid Reusing Needles: Reusing needles increases the risk of infection and dulls the needle, making injections more uncomfortable.
- Safe Disposal of Needles: Dispose of used needles in a designated sharps container, and follow local disposal guidelines to ensure safety.

Handling and Mixing Peptides

If your peptide comes in powder form, it must be reconstituted with sterile water before injection. Proper handling during this process is vital for sterility.

- Use Sterile Water for Injection: Reconstitute peptides using bacteriostatic water (preservative-added sterile water) to maintain sterility.
- Follow Manufacturer Instructions: Follow guidelines for adding the correct amount of water to the peptide vial, and avoid shaking the vial to prevent peptide degradation.
- Store Properly After Reconstitution: Store reconstituted peptides in the refrigerator, and use them within the recommended time frame (usually 30 days) to maintain potency.

4. Safe Storage Practices

Peptides are sensitive to temperature, light, and contamination, so proper storage is essential to preserve their potency and effectiveness.

General Storage Guidelines

- Refrigeration: Most peptides should be stored in the refrigerator to maintain stability, especially after reconstitution. Keep peptides in a designated area of the refrigerator where they won't be exposed to frequent temperature changes.
- Avoid Freezing: While peptides need cool temperatures, freezing them can damage the peptide structure, making them less effective.
- Minimize Light Exposure: Store peptides in their original, opaque containers or in a dark place to protect them from light, which can degrade certain peptides.
- Check Expiration Dates: Always check the expiration dates and discard any peptides that are past their shelf life, as expired peptides may lose efficacy or cause adverse reactions.

Monitoring and Adjusting Based on Feedback

Regularly monitoring your body's response to peptides allows you to make adjustments and optimize your regimen for maximum safety and effectiveness.

- Track Physical and Mental Responses

Keep a record of how you feel each day, noting any side effects, physical changes, or mood shifts. This log provides valuable feedback that can help you adjust dosages or timing based on your body's responses.

Example: Energy levels, sleep quality, muscle recovery, skin changes, mood, and any mild side effects like injection site reactions.

- Schedule Regular Health Check-Ups

Routine check-ups and blood tests help monitor key health markers like hormone levels, liver function, and immune response. These check-ups are particularly important if you're using peptides that affect hormone levels or metabolic function.

- Key Markers to Monitor: Growth hormone levels, blood sugar, liver enzymes, and kidney function for comprehensive health monitoring.
- Consult a Professional: Work with a healthcare provider to review your lab results and adjust your peptide regimen as needed for safe, long-term use.

Key Takeaways for Safe Peptide Usage

1. Follow Proper Dosage and Administration Protocols: Starting with low doses and using the correct administration technique reduces the risk of side effects and improves outcomes.
2. Prioritize Hygiene and Sterility: Clean, safe injection practices and proper handling of reconstituted peptides help prevent infections and irritation.
3. Store Peptides Carefully: Proper storage in a cool, dark place preserves peptide potency and efficacy.

4. Monitor Regularly and Adjust: Keep track of physical and mental responses, adjust dosages as needed, and consult a healthcare provider for periodic check-ups to ensure long-term safety.

6.3 When to Seek Medical Advice

While peptide therapy is generally safe and well-tolerated, knowing when to consult a healthcare provider is essential for ensuring your safety. Seeking medical advice when experiencing unusual symptoms or side effects helps prevent potential complications and allows for any necessary adjustments to your regimen. A proactive approach to health monitoring can make your peptide journey both safer and more effective, giving you the confidence to pursue your anti-aging and wellness goals.

Why Medical Guidance is Important in Peptide Therapy

Peptide therapy is highly individualized, and each person's response to peptides can vary based on factors like health history, lifestyle, and dosage. Having access to a healthcare provider familiar with peptide therapy ensures that you can receive tailored advice and timely support. A provider can offer insights on proper dosages, help monitor health markers, and address any side effects or concerns that arise.

Key benefits of medical guidance include:

1. Personalized Dosage Adjustments: Healthcare providers can assess your progress and adjust peptide dosages to meet

your unique needs, reducing the risk of side effects and enhancing effectiveness.

2. Regular Health Monitoring: Routine check-ups and lab tests allow for the early detection of any health changes, helping you make informed adjustments to your peptide regimen.

3. Expert Advice on Side Effects: Providers can help you distinguish between common, mild side effects and more serious symptoms that may require intervention.

4. Support in Managing Comorbid Conditions: If you have pre-existing health conditions, a provider can help ensure that peptide therapy complements your overall health management plan safely.

Signs and Symptoms That Warrant Medical Advice

While most side effects of peptide therapy are mild and temporary, certain symptoms may indicate the need for medical attention. Understanding these signs helps you know when to consult a provider for guidance and further evaluation.

1. Persistent or Severe Injection Site Reactions

While mild redness, swelling, or tenderness at the injection site is common, persistent or severe reactions may suggest an allergic response or infection.

Signs to Watch For: Persistent pain, swelling, redness, or warmth around the injection site that lasts more than 48 hours, or the appearance of a rash.

Why Seek Advice: These symptoms could indicate an infection or local allergic reaction, both of which may require medical intervention.

Potential Actions: A healthcare provider may recommend an antibiotic ointment or, in rare cases, an oral antibiotic. They may also suggest changing injection sites or adjusting injection technique to minimize irritation.

2. Severe Headaches or Migraines

Mild headaches can sometimes occur with peptides that influence growth hormone release, but severe or persistent headaches are less common and should be evaluated.

Signs to Watch For: Intense, throbbing headaches, sensitivity to light or sound, or accompanying symptoms like nausea or vision changes.

Why Seek Advice: Severe headaches can signal a reaction to dosage or an interaction with other medications. Some peptides may affect fluid balance, which can occasionally lead to increased pressure in the head.

Potential Actions: A provider may recommend reducing the dosage, changing the time of administration, or conducting a blood pressure check to rule out underlying causes.

3. Mood Swings, Anxiety, or Emotional Changes

Peptides that affect hormones, like growth hormone or cortisol, may occasionally lead to mood fluctuations. While mild mood shifts are common, severe or persistent changes should be addressed.

Signs to Watch For: Noticeable irritability, mood swings, heightened anxiety, or feelings of depression that are out of character or last longer than a few days.

Why Seek Advice: Persistent emotional changes may indicate that peptide therapy is impacting hormone levels or neurotransmitters in a way that affects mood. Professional guidance can help determine if dosage adjustments are necessary.

Potential Actions: The provider may recommend reducing the peptide dosage, adjusting the timing, or suggesting complementary therapies for mood stabilization, such as relaxation techniques or lifestyle changes.

4. Persistent Fatigue or Unexplained Weakness

While certain peptides may cause mild drowsiness, persistent fatigue or a noticeable decline in energy may require evaluation, especially if it interferes with daily activities.

Signs to Watch For: Constant tiredness, low energy, difficulty concentrating, or muscle weakness that is not alleviated by rest.

Why Seek Advice: Fatigue can sometimes indicate hormonal imbalances or an interaction between peptides and other medications, particularly if peptides are impacting thyroid or adrenal function.

Potential Actions: The provider may conduct a blood test to check thyroid function, iron levels, and adrenal health, and adjust your peptide regimen based on the results.

5. Rapid Weight Gain or Swelling

Peptides that influence growth hormone levels or metabolism can occasionally lead to water retention, but significant weight gain or swelling may need medical assessment.

Signs to Watch For: Sudden weight gain, noticeable bloating, swelling in the hands, feet, or face, or shortness of breath.
Why Seek Advice: Rapid weight gain or swelling can sometimes indicate fluid retention, hormonal shifts, or, in rare cases, an impact on kidney function.
Potential Actions: A provider may adjust the dosage or recommend additional tests to check for kidney function and electrolyte balance. They may also suggest dietary adjustments to reduce sodium intake.

6. Digestive Issues

Digestive issues are not common with peptides, but some users may experience nausea, upset stomach, or changes in bowel habits, especially with oral peptides.

Signs to Watch For: Persistent nausea, bloating, stomach cramps, or changes in stool consistency lasting more than a few days.
Why Seek Advice: Digestive symptoms may indicate sensitivity to the peptide or an interaction with other supplements or medications.
Potential Actions: The provider may recommend spacing out doses, taking peptides with food, or adjusting the delivery

method (e.g., switching from oral to injectable peptides if feasible).

7. Signs of an Allergic Reaction

Although rare, allergic reactions to peptides can occur. Recognizing the signs and knowing when to seek immediate medical care is essential.

Signs to Watch For: Hives, itching, swelling of the face or throat, difficulty breathing, or a rapid heartbeat.
Why Seek Immediate Medical Attention: Severe allergic reactions require prompt intervention to prevent complications. This type of reaction, known as anaphylaxis, is a medical emergency.
Potential Actions: Call emergency services or go to the nearest emergency room if you suspect a severe allergic reaction. Inform your healthcare provider afterward to discuss alternatives and identify the specific allergen.

Routine Health Monitoring for Long-Term Safety

In addition to being aware of signs and symptoms that warrant medical advice, regular health monitoring provides proactive support for your peptide therapy regimen. Routine check-ups, blood tests, and other health assessments help ensure that peptides are working effectively and safely over the long term.

Recommended Health Assessments for Peptide Users:

1. Blood Tests: Regular blood tests allow you to monitor markers like hormone levels, liver enzymes, kidney function, and blood sugar. These markers provide valuable insights into your body's response to peptides.

2. Bone Density Scans: For individuals using peptides aimed at muscle and joint health, periodic bone density scans help monitor bone health, especially if hormone levels are affected.

3. Skin Health Assessments: For peptides used in skin rejuvenation, regular skin health assessments can track changes in elasticity, hydration, and pigmentation.

Frequency of Monitoring

Initial Assessment: Before starting peptide therapy, get a comprehensive health assessment to establish baseline levels for hormone, liver, and kidney function.

Quarterly or Biannual Check-Ups: Schedule follow-up tests every three to six months to assess your progress and make adjustments to your regimen as needed.

Yearly Health Review: An annual comprehensive health review allows you and your provider to evaluate long-term effects, ensuring that your peptide therapy continues to align with your wellness goals.

Building a Collaborative Relationship with Your Healthcare Provider

Having a supportive healthcare provider who understands peptide therapy is invaluable. Open communication, regular consultations, and shared decision-making enhance the safety and effectiveness of your regimen, giving you peace of mind throughout your journey.

Be Honest About Symptoms: Always share any side effects or changes you notice, even if they seem minor. This transparency allows your provider to make informed decisions and adjust your regimen as needed.

Ask Questions: Don't hesitate to ask questions about dosage, side effects, and potential interactions with other treatments. Understanding your regimen empowers you to make informed choices.

Stay Open to Adjustments: Your provider may suggest changes to dosages, timing, or peptide types based on your progress and health status. Being open to adjustments helps you achieve the best outcomes safely.

Key Takeaways for Seeking Medical Advice in Peptide Therapy

1. Know When to Consult a Provider: Be aware of persistent symptoms or unusual side effects that warrant professional guidance, such as severe headaches, mood changes, or persistent fatigue.

2. Monitor Your Health Regularly: Routine blood tests and health assessments provide proactive support, ensuring peptides are working safely over time.

3. Build a Supportive Provider Relationship: Regular consultations and open communication with a knowledgeable provider enhance the safety and effectiveness of your peptide therapy.

6.4 Creating a Personal Safety Plan

A well-thought-out safety plan is essential for anyone embarking on peptide therapy, as it provides clear guidelines on how to manage dosage, monitor for side effects, and know when to seek medical support. A personal safety plan not only gives you confidence as you progress in your peptide regimen but also allows you to track your response in an organized, proactive way. By structuring your approach to safety, you ensure that you're maximizing benefits while minimizing risks, creating a sustainable foundation for your anti-aging journey.

Why a Personal Safety Plan is Essential

While peptides offer remarkable benefits for anti-aging, health, and vitality, a structured plan ensures that you approach your regimen with caution and care. Having a personal safety plan:

1. Promotes Consistency: A well-organized approach helps you stay consistent, tracking doses and monitoring responses to ensure optimal results.
2. Enhances Self-Awareness: A plan that includes regular self-assessment and symptom tracking allows you to better understand your body's reactions to peptides, helping to prevent unwanted side effects.
3. Prepares for Emergencies: Knowing when and how to seek help in case of unexpected reactions is key to ensuring that any issues are managed quickly and effectively.

4. Provides Guidance and Accountability: A personal safety plan offers a clear framework for your peptide therapy journey, creating a sense of accountability and structure that supports long-term adherence and results.

Step-by-Step Guide to Creating a Personal Safety Plan

A personalized safety plan for peptide therapy involves setting up a structured regimen that includes dosage schedules, tracking methods, symptom monitoring, and access to emergency contacts or healthcare providers. Here's a detailed guide on how to build each component of your plan.

1. Define Your Dosage Schedule and Regimen

Start by establishing a clear dosage schedule, including frequency, timing, and the specific peptides you're using. Keeping track of dosages helps prevent overdosing, missed doses, and inconsistencies that may reduce peptide efficacy or increase side effects.

Set Dosage Goals: Outline the starting dose for each peptide, along with any gradual increases that align with your goals. For example, if you're using a growth hormone-releasing peptide, consider starting with the lowest effective dose and increasing over several weeks as your body adapts.
Create a Schedule: Map out a calendar or use a planner to record each dose, the time of day, and any necessary instructions (e.g., take before bedtime or after a workout).
Keep Dosages Separate if Needed: Some peptides may work best when taken individually, rather than in combination with

others. Include any instructions on separating doses if recommended by your provider.

2. Choose a Tracking Method

Tracking your body's response is a key part of any peptide regimen, helping you to detect patterns, monitor effectiveness, and identify side effects early. A tracking system can be as simple as a journal or as comprehensive as a digital health app.

Journaling: A notebook dedicated to your peptide journey allows you to write daily reflections on physical sensations, mood, energy levels, and any noticeable changes.
Digital Health Apps: Apps designed for health tracking can be used to log doses, set reminders, and record symptoms, making it easier to identify patterns over time.
Weekly Reviews: Set aside time each week to review your entries, looking for any emerging trends or changes in your health markers.

3. Establish Symptom Monitoring Guidelines

While mild side effects are often manageable, certain symptoms require close monitoring to ensure they don't worsen or interfere with daily life. Your safety plan should include a checklist of potential side effects and guidelines for monitoring them.

Identify Common Side Effects: Include a list of common side effects, such as mild headaches, minor injection site irritation, or fatigue, and note when they tend to appear (e.g., shortly after injection).

Track Symptoms Daily: Use a scale of 1-10 to rate any discomfort or symptoms you experience each day, noting the time and any activities that might have influenced these symptoms.

Set Thresholds for Action: Define the point at which a symptom warrants action. For example, if a mild headache becomes persistent or severe, this would trigger a step in your plan, such as reducing the dosage or consulting a provider.

4. Plan for Regular Health Assessments

Routine health assessments allow for a more objective look at how your peptide regimen is affecting your body. Include a timeline for regular check-ups, blood tests, and other necessary screenings in your plan.

Schedule Blood Tests: Regular blood tests can monitor hormone levels, kidney and liver function, and other markers that provide insights into how well your body is responding to peptides.

Check-In Frequency: Depending on your goals and provider recommendations, consider quarterly, biannual, or annual check-ups to review progress and make any necessary adjustments.

Track Key Health Indicators: Include any specific health indicators related to your goals, such as IGF-1 levels for growth hormone support, skin elasticity for anti-aging, or muscle recovery markers for physical fitness.

Establish Emergency Protocols

Part of a comprehensive safety plan involves preparing for rare but possible adverse reactions, ensuring you know when and how to seek medical attention. Emergency protocols offer peace of mind and readiness, should you experience any unexpected reactions to peptides.

Emergency Contacts

Include a list of emergency contacts, such as your primary healthcare provider, a peptide therapy specialist, and a close family member or friend who is familiar with your regimen.

Healthcare Provider Contact: Have the contact information of your primary healthcare provider or peptide specialist on hand for quick consultation if needed.

Family/Friend Contact: Designate a trusted family member or friend who can assist you in case of a sudden reaction, especially if you're experiencing symptoms that limit mobility or cognition.

List of Urgent Symptoms

Create a checklist of urgent symptoms that require immediate medical attention, helping you act quickly if they occur.

Examples of Urgent Symptoms:

- Difficulty breathing or swelling around the face and throat (potential allergic reaction).

- Persistent or severe chest pain, sudden dizziness, or loss of consciousness.

- Persistent pain, warmth, or redness at the injection site that worsens over 48 hours.

Action Steps in Case of Emergency

Outline clear steps to take in the event of an emergency, ensuring that you're prepared to act quickly.

Step 1: Stop taking all peptides immediately if you suspect a serious reaction, and record any symptoms in detail.

Step 2: Contact your healthcare provider or an emergency service for further guidance and inform them about your current peptide regimen.

Step 3: Keep records of any medications or interventions recommended by your provider to share with your primary care team.

Build a Support Network

Having a support network is invaluable for any wellness journey. In addition to medical professionals, consider including friends, family, or even online communities that can offer encouragement, accountability, and advice.

Friends and Family: Share your goals and plans with trusted individuals who can offer support, whether it's a reminder to follow your regimen or a sympathetic ear when discussing progress.

Healthcare Team: Establish a network of healthcare providers, including a primary care physician, any specialists involved in your care, and a pharmacist, if needed.

Online or Local Wellness Groups: Connecting with others who have similar goals or are also using peptide therapy can provide helpful insights, motivation, and shared experiences. Many online forums offer advice on peptide safety and goal-setting.

Reassess and Adjust as Needed

A personal safety plan is a living document that should evolve based on your experiences, responses, and goals. Periodic reassessment ensures that your plan remains relevant and effective, supporting your long-term wellness journey.

Monthly or Quarterly Reviews: Set aside time each month or quarter to evaluate your regimen, symptoms, and progress. This allows you to make adjustments based on new information or changes in your health.

Stay Open to Adjustments: If a particular peptide or dosage isn't producing the desired results, consider discussing alternatives with your healthcare provider. Flexibility helps you refine your approach for continuous improvement.

Celebrate Milestones: Recognize and celebrate small successes in your anti-aging journey. Noticing positive changes in energy, mood, or appearance reinforces your commitment and keeps you motivated to continue.

Key Components of Your Personal Safety Plan

Summarizing your personal safety plan in a checklist can help ensure that all key components are covered, making it easy to reference and follow. Here's an example:

- Dosage and Schedule: Record starting doses, gradual adjustments, and dosing intervals.
- Tracking Method: Choose between journaling, apps, or both for recording symptoms and progress.
- Symptom Monitoring: List common side effects and set threshold levels that trigger action.
- Health Assessments: Schedule regular blood tests and check-ups based on provider recommendations.
- Emergency Protocols: Identify urgent symptoms, emergency contacts, and action steps.
- Support Network: Include healthcare providers, trusted friends or family, and online or local wellness groups.
- Routine Reassessment: Plan monthly or quarterly reviews to assess progress and make necessary adjustments.

Building Confidence in Your Peptide Journey

A personal safety plan provides a structured, proactive approach to peptide therapy, helping you minimize risks, maximize benefits, and stay informed about your health. By following these protocols and guidelines, you're not only supporting a successful anti-aging journey but also fostering a sense of empowerment, allowing you to enjoy the results with confidence and peace of mind. A well-planned peptide regimen, grounded in safety and self-awareness, opens the door to long-term wellness and vitality, making each step of your journey rewarding and enriching.

Chapter 7: Sourcing Quality Peptides and Ensuring Efficacy

7.1 Identifying Trustworthy Peptide Suppliers

When embarking on a peptide therapy journey, sourcing high-quality peptides is essential to ensure safety, efficacy, and consistent results. Trustworthy suppliers provide peptides that are pure, potent, and manufactured to meet rigorous standards. However, the increasing popularity of peptide therapy has led to a surge in suppliers, making it challenging to distinguish reputable sources from those that compromise quality for profit.

Why Quality Sourcing Matters in Peptide Therapy

Peptides are biologically active molecules that require careful handling and precision in manufacturing. Sourcing peptides from a reputable supplier ensures that you're receiving a product that has been tested for purity, potency, and stability. Poorly manufactured peptides can contain contaminants, have inconsistent potency, or degrade quickly, leading to ineffective results or even adverse reactions.

Benefits of sourcing from trusted suppliers include:

1. Assurance of Purity and Potency: Reputable suppliers adhere to high manufacturing standards, ensuring that peptides are free of contaminants and maintain consistent potency.
2. Transparency and Accountability: Trustworthy vendors provide detailed information on their manufacturing processes, testing protocols, and ingredient sourcing.
3. Reliable Customer Support: Reputable suppliers are available to answer questions, provide product information, and address any concerns regarding product quality.
4. Enhanced Safety: Quality peptides reduce the risk of side effects or adverse reactions caused by impurities or inconsistencies.

Key Qualities to Look for in a Peptide Supplier

Choosing a reliable supplier involves assessing several factors, from the source of their ingredients to the quality control measures they have in place. Below are the essential qualities to look for in a peptide supplier.

1. Commitment to Good Manufacturing Practices (GMP)

Good Manufacturing Practices (GMP) are standards that ensure products are consistently produced and controlled according to quality standards. GMP-certified facilities adhere to strict protocols for cleanliness, consistency, and quality control, making this certification an important indicator of a supplier's commitment to safety and efficacy.

What to Look For: Check for a GMP certification or confirmation that the peptides are produced in GMP-certified facilities. Reputable suppliers will typically mention GMP compliance on their website or product descriptions.

Why It Matters: GMP certification helps ensure that peptides are produced in a clean, controlled environment, reducing the risk of contamination and quality inconsistencies.

2. Third-Party Testing and Certificates of Analysis (COA)

Third-party testing involves sending peptide batches to an independent laboratory for analysis, ensuring that the product meets quality standards for purity, potency, and absence of contaminants. A Certificate of Analysis (COA) provides detailed information on the testing results, typically including data on peptide concentration, purity, and any potential impurities.

What to Look For: Choose suppliers that provide a COA for each batch of peptides. The COA should be available on their website or upon request.

Why It Matters: Third-party testing verifies the accuracy of the product's labeling and assures customers that the peptide meets high purity and potency standards. A COA provides transparency and builds trust in the product's quality.

3. Transparency in Ingredient Sourcing

A reputable supplier should be transparent about the sources of their raw ingredients and the locations of their manufacturing facilities. Quality peptide suppliers work with verified sources, whether domestic or international, that follow ethical and sustainable sourcing practices.

What to Look For: Information on where and how raw ingredients are sourced. Suppliers that are committed to transparency may mention partnerships with reliable manufacturers or provide insights into their sourcing practices.
Why It Matters: Knowing the origin of ingredients adds an extra layer of assurance. High-quality, ethically sourced ingredients contribute to the overall efficacy and safety of the peptide product.

4. Positive Customer Reviews and Reputation

Customer reviews provide valuable insights into the reliability and quality of a supplier. Reputable suppliers often have a history of satisfied customers and positive feedback, which can be a strong indicator of trustworthiness.

What to Look For: Look for reviews on the supplier's website, independent review platforms, and industry forums.

Pay attention to feedback regarding product quality, consistency, and customer service.

Why It Matters: Positive reviews from real customers indicate that the supplier consistently provides quality products and reliable service. Look for patterns in reviews, such as mentions of effective results and responsive customer support.

5. Clear and Accessible Contact Information

Reliable suppliers should have accessible contact information, allowing customers to ask questions, request documentation, or discuss any concerns. A legitimate company will typically provide a business address, phone number, email, and possibly a live chat feature on their website.

What to Look For: An active phone number, email address, and physical business address. Some suppliers may also have customer service representatives available for real-time support.

Why It Matters: Accessible contact information demonstrates accountability and customer support. It reassures customers that they can reach out if they encounter any issues with their purchase.

Red Flags to Avoid When Choosing a Peptide Supplier

While many suppliers offer high-quality peptides, some vendors cut corners or prioritize profit over product safety and efficacy. Being aware of common red flags can help you avoid unreliable suppliers and protect your health.

1. Lack of Transparency

If a supplier doesn't provide information on their manufacturing process, ingredient sourcing, or testing practices, it's a warning sign. Reputable suppliers are transparent about how their products are made and are willing to share relevant information with customers.

Signs to Watch For: Vague or missing information on the website about ingredient sources, manufacturing practices, or testing protocols. Lack of a Certificate of Analysis for each batch.

Why It's a Red Flag: Lack of transparency can indicate low-quality manufacturing practices or shortcuts in quality control, increasing the risk of contaminated or inconsistent products.

2. Too-Good-To-Be-True Pricing

Quality peptide manufacturing is a costly process that involves stringent quality control, specialized equipment, and high-quality raw ingredients. Extremely low prices may indicate poor manufacturing practices or lower-quality ingredients.

Signs to Watch For: Prices significantly lower than other reputable suppliers or frequent, steep discounts that seem unsustainable.

Why It's a Red Flag: Cheap pricing often correlates with compromises in quality, such as lower purity, unregulated sourcing, or lack of testing. Paying slightly more for peptides from reputable suppliers can provide peace of mind and better results.

3. Poor Customer Reviews and Complaints

Negative reviews or unresolved complaints about product quality, consistency, or customer service can signal issues with the supplier. Reputable companies work hard to resolve customer issues and are responsive to feedback.

Signs to Watch For: Multiple complaints about product quality, inconsistent effects, or lack of customer support. Pay attention to patterns, especially if several reviews mention similar concerns.
Why It's a Red Flag: A history of negative feedback may suggest unreliable quality control, unresponsive customer service, or other issues that could affect the safety and efficacy of the product.

4. No Third-Party Testing or COA

Reputable suppliers conduct third-party testing to verify purity and potency, and they make this information accessible to customers. If a supplier does not offer a **Certificate of Analysis** or refuses to provide one upon request, it's best to look elsewhere.

Signs to Watch For: No mention of third-party testing or lack of available COAs for specific batches.

Why It's a Red Flag: Third-party testing is crucial for verifying product quality. A lack of testing information raises questions about the authenticity and purity of the peptides.

5. Lack of Clear Refund or Return Policy

A reputable supplier stands behind their products and offers a clear refund or return policy. If a company has a vague or restrictive return policy, it may be a sign that they're unwilling to take responsibility for their products.

Signs to Watch For: No refund or return policy, restrictive conditions, or lack of clarity about how returns are processed. **Why It's a Red Flag:** A transparent return policy reflects confidence in product quality and ensures that customers have recourse if they are unsatisfied with their purchase.

Steps for Verifying Product Authenticity

Once you've selected a supplier, taking a few extra steps to verify product authenticity helps confirm that you're receiving a genuine, high-quality product. Here's how to verify that your peptides meet the standards promised by the supplier.

1. Request a Certificate of Analysis (COA)

Ask for a COA specific to the batch you're purchasing. The COA should include details on purity, concentration, and any tests for contaminants, providing assurance that the product is accurately labeled.

What to Look For: Confirm that the COA is from an independent, accredited laboratory and includes the peptide's concentration, purity percentage, and test date.

Why It Matters: A COA verifies that the peptide has been tested for quality and that the supplier's claims are backed by data.

2. Check Product Packaging and Labels

Packaging and labeling can provide clues about product quality and authenticity. Quality suppliers invest in professional packaging that protects the product from contamination and includes clear, accurate labels.

What to Look For: Ensure that the packaging is tamper-proof, includes clear instructions, and lists the expiration date. Some products may have batch numbers or QR codes that link to more information.

Why It Matters: Proper packaging preserves peptide potency and minimizes the risk of contamination, ensuring a safe and effective product.

3. Test the Peptides at a Trusted Laboratory

For added peace of mind, you may consider sending a small sample of the peptide to an independent lab for testing, especially if you're using peptides for long-term or intensive therapies.

What to Look For: Request tests for purity and potency. Some labs also offer contaminant testing for added safety.

Why It Matters: Third-party testing provides an unbiased confirmation of product quality, helping to ensure that you're receiving the expected concentration and purity.

4. Monitor Initial Effects and Adjust Accordingly

Once you begin using the peptide, carefully monitor your body's response and any physical changes. High-quality peptides generally produce noticeable effects within a few weeks, depending on the type and purpose.

What to Look For: Track specific markers based on your goals, such as improved skin elasticity, muscle recovery, or energy levels. Compare your experiences with typical expected results for that peptide.
Why It Matters: Monitoring initial effects helps confirm that the peptide is effective and consistent with the claims made by the supplier.

Chapter 7: Sourcing Quality Peptides and Ensuring Efficacy

7.2 How to Evaluate Product Quality

Evaluating the quality of peptides is crucial for achieving safe, effective results from your anti-aging or wellness regimen. With the rising popularity of peptide therapy, it's more important than ever to assess product quality and ensure you're purchasing from a reputable supplier. A high-quality peptide is marked by purity, stability, accurate labeling, and adherence to rigorous manufacturing standards, while a poor-quality product may be contaminated, less potent, or even counterfeit.

Why Product Quality Matters in Peptide Therapy

Peptides are biologically active molecules that require precision in manufacturing and handling to maintain their potency and safety. High-quality peptides work effectively with your body, supporting functions like collagen production, muscle repair, and immune resilience. In contrast, low-quality or counterfeit peptides may not only be ineffective but also carry health risks.

Key reasons to prioritize quality in peptide selection include:

1. Consistent Results: Pure, potent peptides provide reliable outcomes, helping you achieve your health and anti-aging goals.
2. Reduced Risk of Side Effects: Quality peptides are free from contaminants and impurities, minimizing the risk of adverse reactions.
3. Optimal Efficacy: Well-made peptides maintain their structure and function, ensuring that they deliver the intended benefits without degradation.
4. Safety Assurance: Reputable manufacturers adhere to standards that ensure the product's safety, giving you peace of mind in your therapy regimen.

Steps to Evaluate Peptide Quality

Evaluating peptide quality involves checking for specific characteristics that indicate purity, potency, and authenticity. By following these steps, you can make informed choices that prioritize safety and efficacy.

1. Assess the Physical Appearance and Packaging

The physical appearance and packaging of a peptide product can provide valuable insights into its quality. While appearance alone doesn't guarantee quality, certain characteristics often indicate whether the peptide has been handled and stored correctly.

Powder Form and Color: High-quality peptides are usually provided as a white, lyophilized (freeze-dried) powder. The powder should be uniformly white and free from discoloration or clumping. Discoloration or unusual texture can suggest improper storage or contamination.

Absence of Residue or Foreign Particles: Inspect the vial for any visible particles or residue. The peptide powder should be clean, with no visible particles or inconsistencies.

Proper Labeling: Look for clear, professional labeling on the product. The label should include the peptide's name, concentration, expiration date, and storage instructions. Clear labeling reflects the manufacturer's attention to detail and commitment to transparency.

Tamper-Proof Seals: High-quality products come with tamper-proof seals, which prevent contamination and signal that the product hasn't been altered since leaving the manufacturer.

Red Flags in Appearance and Packaging

Be cautious of peptides that display the following characteristics, as they may indicate low-quality or improperly handled products:

Discoloration: Yellowish or brownish color can signal contamination or degradation, reducing the peptide's effectiveness.

Visible Residue or Foreign Particles: Any visible particles or residue within the vial could indicate poor manufacturing practices or contamination.

Lack of Professional Packaging: Poor labeling, absence of an expiration date, or missing storage instructions are signs of a potentially low-quality product.

2. Verify Third-Party Testing and Certificates of Analysis (COA)

One of the most reliable ways to evaluate peptide quality is through third-party testing and a Certificate of Analysis (COA). A COA provides objective, laboratory-confirmed information about the peptide's purity, concentration, and absence of contaminants, helping you make informed purchasing decisions.

Purity Percentage: High-quality peptides should have a purity level of at least 95-99%, as indicated on the COA. Purity reflects the percentage of the product that is the desired peptide, with the remainder typically being residual moisture or benign stabilizers.

Concentration Consistency: The COA should indicate the concentration of the peptide, confirming that it aligns with the label. Consistency in concentration ensures that you're receiving an accurate dose for effective results.

Testing for Contaminants: A reputable COA includes testing results for potential contaminants, such as heavy metals,

solvents, or microbial impurities. These contaminants can compromise both the safety and effectiveness of the peptide.
Date of Testing: Check the date on the COA to ensure it's recent and relevant to the batch you're purchasing. A recent COA indicates that the peptide's quality was verified shortly before it was made available to consumers.

How to Access and Interpret a COA

Most reputable suppliers provide COAs on their website or make them available upon request. When reviewing a COA:
1. Confirm Authenticity: Ensure that the COA comes from an independent, accredited laboratory, not from the manufacturer's in-house testing.
2. Look for Comprehensive Testing Information: The COA should include purity, concentration, and contaminant testing, providing a full profile of the peptide's quality.
3. Check Batch Numbers: The COA should reference a specific batch number, which you can match to the product you're purchasing to confirm that the testing applies to your specific peptide.

3. Evaluate the Supplier's Manufacturing Standards

Understanding the manufacturing standards of your peptide supplier can provide further assurance of product quality. Reputable manufacturers follow rigorous protocols, such as Good Manufacturing Practices (GMP), which ensure consistency, cleanliness, and quality control throughout the production process.

Good Manufacturing Practices (GMP) Compliance: Suppliers that follow GMP are committed to producing peptides in a controlled, sanitary environment. GMP-certified facilities must meet specific criteria for cleanliness, quality control, and employee training.

Adherence to Pharmaceutical-Grade Standards: Pharmaceutical-grade peptides are produced to higher standards than research-grade peptides, focusing on both purity and consistency. Look for suppliers who mention pharmaceutical-grade standards if you're using peptides for health and wellness purposes.

Sterility Assurance: Sterility is especially critical for peptides intended for injection. Ensure that the manufacturing process includes sterilization protocols, which reduce the risk of contamination and infection.

4. Examine Labeling Accuracy and Product Information

Accurate labeling is essential for evaluating peptide quality, as it confirms the concentration, storage instructions, and usage guidelines. Detailed, accurate labeling reflects a supplier's commitment to transparency and quality assurance.

Concentration and Dosage Information: The label should clearly indicate the peptide's concentration, typically in milligrams (mg) per vial. Accurate concentration information allows you to measure doses precisely.

Storage Instructions: Quality peptides come with clear storage instructions, often requiring refrigeration to preserve stability. Adhering to these guidelines prevents peptide degradation, ensuring effectiveness.

Expiration Date: An expiration date is essential for gauging the peptide's shelf life. Quality peptides retain their potency until the expiration date if stored properly.

5. Evaluate Customer Reviews and Testimonials

Customer feedback provides valuable insights into a product's effectiveness and consistency. While reviews alone cannot guarantee quality, they offer a glimpse into the experiences of other users, helping you gauge whether the supplier delivers reliable products.

Focus on Consistency and Effectiveness: Look for patterns in reviews that mention consistent effects, reliable dosages, and positive results. Consistency in effectiveness is a good indicator of high-quality peptides.

Consider Feedback on Customer Support: A supplier's customer support reflects their commitment to customer satisfaction. Positive feedback on support availability, responsiveness, and willingness to address issues is a reassuring sign.

Cross-Check on Independent Review Sites: To get an unbiased view, check reviews on independent platforms or forums where peptide users share their experiences.

Practical Tips for Evaluating Product Quality at Home

Once you've received your peptide product, a few practical steps can help confirm that the peptide meets quality standards. While these evaluations don't replace professional testing, they provide additional assurance.

1. Inspect for Tampering and Packaging Integrity

Inspect the packaging for any signs of tampering or damage that may indicate compromised quality. Quality suppliers use tamper-proof seals, shrink-wrap, or security labels to protect the product.

Check for Broken Seals: If the seal is broken or damaged, contact the supplier for clarification. A broken seal may indicate tampering or mishandling during shipping.

Examine Packaging Condition: Ensure that the vial and packaging are free from cracks, leaks, or other signs of physical damage that could impact the peptide's integrity.

2. Observe Product Stability After Reconstitution

Many peptides require reconstitution (mixing with sterile water) before use. Once reconstituted, observe the peptide for any unexpected changes in appearance.

Look for Dissolution Clarity: After reconstitution, the solution should be clear, without any cloudiness or particles. Cloudiness can indicate instability, which may reduce the peptide's effectiveness.

Monitor for Color Changes: The solution should remain clear after mixing. Any yellowing or discoloration may indicate contamination or instability.

3. Store Peptides Correctly for Long-Term Stability

Proper storage is essential for maintaining peptide potency. Most peptides should be refrigerated after reconstitution to prevent degradation.

Check the Temperature: Store peptides at the temperature recommended on the label, typically between 2-8°C (36-46°F). Avoid freezing, as this can damage the peptide structure.

Minimize Light Exposure: Store peptides in a dark place, away from direct sunlight, which can degrade certain compounds and reduce potency.

7.3 Storage and Handling for Maximum Potency

Proper storage and handling of peptides are essential for maintaining their potency, stability, and safety. Peptides are sensitive molecules that can degrade if exposed to light, heat, moisture, or improper handling. When stored correctly, peptides retain their structure and effectiveness, ensuring that you receive the full therapeutic benefits from each dose.

Why Storage and Handling Matter for Peptide Potency

Peptides are biologically active molecules with delicate structures. Exposure to unfavorable conditions can cause peptides to denature (lose their shape) or degrade, reducing their effectiveness or making them unusable. Proper storage and handling prevent degradation, ensuring that each dose delivers its intended benefits. Key reasons to prioritize correct storage include:

1. Preservation of Potency: Proper storage helps maintain the peptide's strength and effectiveness, allowing you to achieve consistent results with each use.

2. Reduction of Contamination Risks: Following sterile handling procedures minimizes the risk of bacterial or fungal contamination, which is especially important for injectable peptides.

3. Safety Assurance: Quality storage and handling reduce the risk of adverse reactions by preventing peptide degradation or contamination.

4. Cost-Effectiveness: Correct storage practices prevent waste by extending the shelf life of your peptides, ensuring that you get the most value from your investment.

Best Practices for Storing Peptides

Peptides are sensitive to environmental factors like temperature, light, and moisture. Following specific storage guidelines ensures that your peptides remain stable and effective for the duration of their shelf life.

1. Store Peptides in a Cool Environment

Temperature control is one of the most important aspects of peptide storage. Most peptides should be kept in the refrigerator, ideally at a temperature between 2-8°C (36-46°F). Freezing is generally not recommended, as extreme cold can damage peptide structures and reduce efficacy.

Refrigeration: Store peptides in the refrigerator, away from the door, to minimize exposure to temperature fluctuations. The center of the refrigerator is typically the most stable area.

Avoid Freezing: While some peptides may tolerate freezing, many can lose potency or become unstable when frozen. Unless specified by the supplier, avoid freezing peptides.

Keep Away from Heat Sources: Avoid storing peptides near heat sources like stovetops, ovens, or direct sunlight, which can accelerate degradation.

2. Protect Peptides from Light Exposure

Exposure to light can degrade peptides over time, especially if they are stored in transparent or semi-transparent vials. To prevent light damage, store peptides in their original, opaque packaging or in a dark location.

Use Opaque Vials: Many suppliers package peptides in amber or black vials to reduce light exposure. Keep peptides in these vials and avoid transferring them to clear containers.

Refrigerator Placement: If your refrigerator has a transparent door, store peptides in a drawer or compartment that blocks light. Light can penetrate the refrigerator door, especially if it is opened frequently.

Use Dark Storage Bags: Consider placing peptide vials in small, dark storage bags for added protection against light, especially if you are storing multiple vials in the same space.

3. Minimize Exposure to Moisture

Moisture can affect the stability of peptides, especially if they are in powder form before reconstitution. Keeping peptides dry before reconstitution is essential for maintaining potency.

Avoid Humid Storage Areas: Store peptides in a low-humidity environment, away from areas like the bathroom or kitchen, where moisture levels fluctuate.

Reconstitute with Care: When reconstituting peptides, avoid exposing the powder to excess moisture or handling it in a humid environment. Consider using a sterile, dry syringe to ensure precision and avoid contamination.

Proper Handling Techniques for Peptide Stability

In addition to storage, handling practices play a crucial role in maintaining peptide stability. Following these techniques helps preserve peptide structure, potency, and safety.

1. Reconstitute Peptides Carefully

Many peptides come in a lyophilized (freeze-dried) powder form and require reconstitution with a sterile solution, such as bacteriostatic water. Proper reconstitution practices help avoid contamination and ensure that the peptide dissolves completely.

Use Sterile Water for Injection: Bacteriostatic water is commonly recommended for reconstitution, as it contains a preservative (usually benzyl alcohol) that inhibits bacterial growth. This solution is especially useful for peptides that will be stored for more than a few days after reconstitution.

Avoid Shaking the Vial: After adding the sterile water to the vial, gently swirl the vial to dissolve the powder completely.

Shaking can cause peptide degradation, so it's best to avoid this method.

Use the Correct Amount of Solvent: Follow the supplier's guidelines on the amount of solvent needed for reconstitution. Using too little or too much solvent can impact dosage accuracy and efficacy.

2. Practice Sterile Injection Techniques

If you're administering peptides via injection, sterile handling is crucial to prevent contamination and infection. Practicing safe injection techniques protects both the product and your health.

Use a New, Sterile Needle for Each Injection: Avoid reusing needles, as this increases the risk of contamination and can introduce bacteria into the vial.

Disinfect the Injection Site: Clean the injection site with an alcohol swab before administering the peptide to prevent infection.

Store Reconstituted Peptides in the Refrigerator: After reconstitution, peptides should be refrigerated to maintain stability. Many reconstituted peptides are stable for up to 30 days under refrigeration, though this can vary by peptide.

3. Handle Peptides with Clean, Dry Hands

Peptide vials are best handled with clean, dry hands to prevent contamination. Oils, dirt, or moisture on your hands can introduce contaminants to the peptide vial, impacting quality and safety.

Wash Hands Thoroughly: Wash your hands with soap and water before handling peptide vials or reconstituting peptides. Dry them completely to prevent moisture transfer.

Use Gloves if Necessary: If you are handling multiple vials or reconstituting peptides in a non-sterile environment, consider wearing sterile gloves to prevent contamination.

Storing Reconstituted Peptides for Maximum Stability

Reconstituted peptides require specific storage conditions to maintain their potency over time. Following these guidelines helps extend the shelf life and efficacy of your peptides after they've been reconstituted.

1. Keep Reconstituted Peptides Refrigerated

Most reconstituted peptides should be kept in the refrigerator, as low temperatures help preserve their molecular structure and prevent degradation.

Store at 2-8°C (36-46°F): This temperature range is ideal for maintaining peptide stability after reconstitution. If traveling, use a portable cooler to keep peptides within this range.

Monitor the Refrigerator Temperature: Fluctuations in temperature can impact peptide stability. Check your refrigerator periodically to ensure it maintains a consistent temperature.

Avoid Freezing: Reconstituted peptides are generally sensitive to freezing temperatures. Freezing can cause peptides to break down or become less effective.

2. Limit the Time Peptides are Outside the Refrigerator

While administering peptides or preparing doses, limit the amount of time the vial spends outside the refrigerator. Extended exposure to room temperature can lead to peptide degradation, especially in warmer environments.

Prepare Doses Quickly: Minimize the time between removing the peptide vial from the refrigerator and administering the dose. Avoid leaving the vial at room temperature for extended periods.

Return to Refrigerator Immediately: Once you've drawn the required dose, return the vial to the refrigerator promptly to maintain stability.

3. Discard Peptides After the Recommended Period

Reconstituted peptides have a limited shelf life, typically around 2-4 weeks, depending on the peptide and storage conditions. Discarding peptides after their expiration ensures that you're using a potent, safe product.

Follow Shelf Life Guidelines: Each peptide has a recommended storage duration after reconstitution, usually provided by the supplier. Adhere to these guidelines to avoid using degraded peptides.

Check for Signs of Degradation: Before each use, inspect reconstituted peptides for any changes in color, clarity, or consistency. Discoloration or cloudiness can indicate degradation, and such peptides should be discarded.

Common Storage and Handling Mistakes to Avoid

Knowing what to avoid can be as important as knowing what to do. Here are common storage and handling mistakes that can compromise peptide quality and safety:

Leaving Peptides at Room Temperature for Extended Periods: Prolonged exposure to room temperature can cause peptides to degrade. Always store peptides in the refrigerator when not in use.

Using Contaminated Needles or Equipment: Reusing needles or using unsterile equipment increases the risk of contamination, especially for injectable peptides. Use new, sterile needles and syringes each time.

Shaking the Vial During Reconstitution: Shaking can cause peptide degradation. Instead, gently swirl or roll the vial to dissolve the powder fully.

Ignoring Expiration Dates: Using peptides past their expiration date or recommended storage period reduces efficacy and can increase the risk of adverse reactions.

7.4 Avoiding Scams and Choosing the Right Sources

In the world of peptide therapy, the rise in demand has also led to an increase in scams, low-quality products, and unreliable vendors. Choosing the right source for your peptides is vital for ensuring safety, effectiveness, and a positive experience. By understanding the tactics scammers use, recognizing reputable suppliers, and verifying product authenticity, you can confidently source quality peptides that support your anti-aging and wellness goals.

The Risks of Purchasing from Unreliable Sources

Purchasing peptides from untrustworthy sources can lead to various risks, including exposure to contaminated products, inconsistent results, and even legal issues. Low-quality peptides may contain impurities, mislabeled ingredients, or incorrect dosages, compromising both safety and efficacy. Understanding these risks reinforces the importance of selecting a reputable supplier.

Key risks associated with purchasing from unreliable sources include:

1. Health Hazards: Contaminated or impure peptides can introduce harmful substances into the body, leading to infections, allergic reactions, or adverse side effects.

2. Reduced Efficacy: Poor-quality peptides may be less potent or even ineffective, preventing you from achieving desired results and wasting your investment.

3. Legal Complications: Some online vendors sell peptides without proper regulatory compliance, which can lead to legal issues if the products are not approved or labeled correctly.

4. Financial Loss: Purchasing from unreliable sources can result in financial loss if the products do not meet expectations, require frequent replacement, or are not safe for use.

Steps to Avoid Peptide Scams

Avoiding scams requires a careful approach to product selection and supplier verification. By staying vigilant, you can protect yourself from low-quality products and deceptive marketing tactics.

1. Be Cautious of Extremely Low Prices

While it's natural to seek competitive pricing, unusually low prices are often a red flag for scams. High-quality peptide production involves advanced manufacturing techniques, testing, and compliance, making extremely low prices unlikely without compromising quality.

Red Flag: If a supplier's prices are significantly lower than the industry average, they may be cutting corners on quality or selling counterfeit products.

Tips: Compare prices across multiple reputable suppliers to get a sense of the typical cost for high-quality peptides. If a price seems too good to be true, it probably is.

2. Verify Supplier Credentials and Industry Reputation

A reputable supplier will have an established presence in the peptide industry, with verifiable credentials and a positive reputation. Researching the supplier's background, certifications, and customer reviews provides insights into their reliability.

Look for Certifications: Check for Good Manufacturing Practices (GMP) certification, third-party testing, and adherence to pharmaceutical-grade standards. These credentials reflect a commitment to quality and safety.

Read Independent Reviews: Customer reviews on independent websites or forums are often more honest and detailed than those on the supplier's site. Look for patterns in reviews that mention product consistency, effectiveness, and customer service.

Industry Forums: Trusted online forums for peptide users often have threads that discuss reputable suppliers. Engaging in these communities can provide firsthand recommendations and warnings.

3. Avoid Suppliers with Poor or Limited Online Presence

Reputable suppliers maintain a professional online presence, including a well-designed website, clear product information, and responsive customer support. Be cautious of vendors with minimal information, poor website design, or lack of clear contact details.

Red Flags: Websites with broken links, spelling errors, or vague product descriptions may indicate a lack of professionalism. Similarly, a lack of contact information or customer support options is a warning sign.

Tips: Look for suppliers with a clear About Us page, professional website design, and accessible contact information, such as a business address, phone number, and email. Legitimate suppliers often have live chat or customer service representatives available for inquiries.

4. Be Wary of Suppliers Without Third-Party Testing and COAs

Third-party testing is essential for ensuring the purity, potency, and safety of peptides. Reliable suppliers provide a Certificate of Analysis (COA) that verifies the product's quality, confirming that it has been tested for contaminants and meets industry standards.

Red Flag: If a supplier does not provide a COA or seems hesitant to share it, they may be selling untested or low-quality peptides.

Tips: Always request a COA before purchasing, and verify that it comes from an independent, accredited lab. Check the COA for information on purity, concentration, and the date of testing to confirm that it applies to the batch you're purchasing.

5. Avoid Suppliers with Unrealistic Claims or Aggressive Marketing

Scammers often use exaggerated claims or aggressive marketing tactics to attract buyers. Claims of "miracle cures" or "guaranteed results" are usually signs of deceptive marketing, as reputable suppliers avoid making unrealistic promises about peptide benefits.

Red Flag: Statements like "instant results," "no side effects," or "miracle anti-aging" are often used to mislead customers and are not supported by scientific evidence.

Tips: Choose suppliers that provide balanced, fact-based information about their products, including realistic timelines and potential side effects. Reputable suppliers focus on scientific support rather than hype.

Guidelines for Choosing Reputable Peptide Suppliers

After identifying the red flags associated with unreliable vendors, follow these guidelines to find reputable suppliers who prioritize quality, safety, and customer satisfaction.

1. Look for Transparent Product Information and Labeling

Trustworthy suppliers provide detailed product information, including concentration, usage instructions, expiration dates, and storage guidelines. Accurate labeling and transparency are essential for ensuring you're using the product safely and effectively.

What to Look For: Each product should have clear labels with concentration (e.g., mg per vial), recommended usage, and reconstitution instructions. Expiration dates should be visible on the packaging.

Tips: Choose suppliers who make labeling information accessible both on the product and on their website. Reputable suppliers understand the importance of transparency and aim to educate their customers.

2. Check for Good Manufacturing Practices (GMP) Certification

Good Manufacturing Practices (GMP) certification is a quality standard that ensures products are manufactured in a controlled, sanitary environment. GMP certification indicates that the supplier follows strict protocols for consistency, quality control, and safety.

What to Look For: Suppliers should mention GMP compliance on their website or product descriptions. A GMP-certified facility adheres to high standards of cleanliness, quality control, and employee training.

Tips: Prioritize GMP-certified suppliers for peace of mind that the product has been produced according to established safety and quality guidelines.

3. Choose Suppliers with Established Customer Support

Quality suppliers offer reliable customer support to assist with inquiries, product concerns, and order issues. Responsive customer service reflects a supplier's commitment to customer satisfaction and accountability.

What to Look For: Reputable suppliers typically provide multiple contact methods, including phone, email, and live chat. Check for positive feedback on customer support in online reviews.

Tips: Before making a purchase, consider reaching out to customer support with any questions. Their responsiveness and professionalism can give you insights into their dedication to service.

4. Research Supplier Background and Industry Affiliations

Suppliers with industry affiliations or memberships in professional organizations often have a stronger commitment to quality standards. Background research on the supplier's history, certifications, and affiliations adds another layer of confidence in your purchase.

What to Look For: Look for affiliations with industry organizations, positive mentions on trusted forums, and a solid track record in the peptide industry.

Tips: A supplier with a strong reputation in the industry, often backed by affiliations, demonstrates a commitment to meeting standards and maintaining credibility.

Practical Tips for Verifying Product Authenticity

Even after selecting a reputable supplier, taking a few extra steps to verify product authenticity can help ensure that you're receiving genuine, high-quality peptides.

1. Request a Batch-Specific Certificate of Analysis (COA)

A batch-specific COA confirms that the exact batch of peptides you're purchasing has been tested for purity, potency, and contaminants. Reviewing this certificate helps verify that the peptide meets the manufacturer's quality claims.

Steps: Contact customer support to request a COA for the batch associated with your product. Check that the COA includes data on purity, concentration, and testing dates.
Why It's Important: A batch-specific COA confirms that the product has undergone quality checks, reducing the risk of receiving a subpar or counterfeit product.

2. Inspect Packaging and Labeling for Quality

Authentic peptides come in professional packaging with tamper-proof seals, clear labels, and detailed product information. Poor packaging or incomplete labeling can be a sign of a counterfeit or low-quality product.
What to Look For: Ensure that the product has a tamper-proof seal, accurate labeling with concentration and expiration dates, and proper storage instructions.
Tips: Contact the supplier if there are any inconsistencies in the packaging or labeling, and do not use the product if the seal is broken.

3. Test Initial Effects and Monitor for Consistency

Once you start using the peptide, monitor your body's response to confirm that it matches typical effects. High-quality peptides produce consistent, predictable results, while counterfeit or low-quality products may be less effective or cause unusual side effects.

What to Track: Keep a log of your dosage, effects, and any side effects. Compare these to the expected benefits of the peptide to determine consistency and effectiveness.

Why It's Important: Tracking helps you detect any discrepancies early on, allowing you to address issues with the supplier or adjust your regimen if needed.

Chapter 8: Quick Reference Guides and Tools

8.1 Peptide Cheat Sheet – Benefits and Best Practices

A peptide cheat sheet serves as a quick-reference guide for understanding the core benefits, applications, and best practices associated with each peptide in your regimen. With so many peptides available, each with distinct effects on skin, muscle, immunity, and overall wellness, a concise overview of each peptide's key functions and usage recommendations provides a practical tool for both beginners and seasoned users.

Understanding Peptide Benefits and Their Applications

Peptides are short chains of amino acids that act as signaling molecules in the body, helping regulate various biological processes. Different peptides target specific functions, such as skin rejuvenation, muscle growth, immune support, and cognitive enhancement. Here's a breakdown of popular peptides, organized by their primary applications and benefits.

1. Peptides for Skin Health and Anti-Aging

These peptides focus on enhancing skin elasticity, reducing fine lines, and promoting a youthful appearance. They stimulate collagen production, improve skin hydration, and protect against environmental damage.

- **GHK-Cu (Copper Peptide)**

Benefits: Promotes skin elasticity, reduces fine lines, enhances wound healing, and boosts collagen production.

Best Practices: Apply topically as part of a skincare routine or use in subcutaneous injections. Store reconstituted peptides in the refrigerator to preserve potency.

Usage Tips: GHK-Cu is particularly effective when applied at night, as it supports the skin's natural repair process during sleep. Use a low concentration initially to test for skin sensitivity.

- **Matrixyl (Palmitoyl Pentapeptide-4)**

Benefits: Reduces the appearance of wrinkles, improves skin texture, and supports collagen synthesis.

Best Practices: Found in many skincare products, Matrixyl can be used as part of a daily topical regimen. Store in a cool, dark place to maintain stability.

Usage Tips: Apply in the morning and evening after cleansing for best results. Matrixyl pairs well with hyaluronic acid to maximize skin hydration.

- **Argireline (Acetyl Hexapeptide-8)**

Benefits: Reduces fine lines, especially around the eyes and forehead, by relaxing facial muscles.

Best Practices: Apply topically in small amounts, focusing on areas prone to wrinkles. Store at room temperature, away from sunlight.

Usage Tips: Often called ***"Botox in a bottle,"*** Argireline is ideal for targeting expression lines. Use sparingly to prevent over-relaxation of muscles.

2. Peptides for Muscle Growth and Recovery

Muscle-targeting peptides are commonly used in fitness and bodybuilding, as they support growth hormone release, improve muscle tone, and accelerate recovery.

- **CJC-1295 + Ipamorelin**

Benefits: Stimulates growth hormone release, enhances muscle growth, aids in fat loss, and improves recovery.

Best Practices: Administer via subcutaneous injection, typically in cycles (e.g., 6-8 weeks on, 2-4 weeks off). Store in the refrigerator to maintain stability.

Usage Tips: To maximize growth hormone pulses, administer at night on an empty stomach. Pairing with a balanced diet and exercise enhances results.

- **BPC-157 (Body Protective Compound)**

Benefits: Promotes muscle recovery, reduces inflammation, supports joint health, and accelerates wound healing.

Best Practices: Can be administered via injection for targeted areas or taken orally for systemic effects. Refrigerate after reconstitution.

Usage Tips: Ideal for individuals recovering from injuries or looking to reduce joint pain, BPC-157 can be used in combination with physical therapy for faster recovery.

- **TB-500 (Thymosin Beta-4)**

Benefits: Enhances muscle recovery, reduces inflammation, and promotes healing of connective tissues.

Best Practices: Administer via subcutaneous or intramuscular injection. Store refrigerated to maintain potency.

Usage Tips: TB-500 is most effective when administered in cycles, especially for athletes needing quick recovery from training-related injuries.

3. Peptides for Immune Support and Longevity

These peptides are designed to boost immunity, support cellular health, and potentially extend lifespan by improving the body's resilience.

- Epitalon

Benefits: Supports telomere repair, promotes longevity, enhances sleep quality, and boosts immunity.

Best Practices: Administer as an intranasal spray or via injection. Store refrigerated, especially after reconstitution.

Usage Tips: Often used in anti-aging protocols, Epitalon is commonly administered in short cycles (e.g., twice annually) to optimize cellular health.

- **Thymosin Alpha-1**

Benefits: Boosts immune response, supports antiviral and antibacterial defenses, and enhances overall immune resilience.

Best Practices: Administer via subcutaneous injection. Store reconstituted peptides in the refrigerator.

Usage Tips: Ideal during periods of immune vulnerability, Thymosin Alpha-1 can be used preventatively or as a supportive therapy during illness.

4. Peptides for Cognitive Health and Mood Enhancement

Peptides that influence neurochemistry and cognitive function can support mental clarity, enhance focus, and even improve mood. They're often used in conjunction with healthy lifestyle practices for best results.

- **Selank**

Benefits: Reduces anxiety, improves focus, enhances memory, and promotes mental clarity.

Best Practices: Often administered intranasally or via subcutaneous injection. Store in a cool, dark place to maintain stability.

Usage Tips: Selank is particularly beneficial during high-stress periods. It may take a few weeks to experience full effects, so use consistently for best results.

- **Semax**

Benefits: Enhances memory, improves cognitive function, supports neuroprotection, and can boost mood.

Best Practices: Administer intranasally for direct absorption. Keep refrigerated to maintain stability and potency.

Usage Tips: Semax is ideal for those seeking cognitive support, particularly for tasks requiring mental endurance. Administer in small doses initially to assess tolerance.

General Best Practices for Peptide Usage

Alongside individual peptide-specific guidelines, a few general best practices can help optimize the benefits and safety of your peptide therapy. Following these principles ensures you get the most from each peptide while minimizing potential risks.

1. Start with Low Dosages and Gradually Increase

Starting with a low dose allows your body to adapt to peptides, minimizing the risk of side effects. Gradually increasing the dosage ensures that you're safely maximizing the benefits.

Begin with the Minimum Effective Dose: Start with the lowest recommended dose for your specific peptide, then adjust based on your body's response.

Monitor for Side Effects: Track any initial responses, including changes in mood, energy, or physical sensations. If you experience side effects, consider lowering the dose and consulting a healthcare provider if symptoms persist.

2. Use Peptides in Cycles to Prevent Tolerance

Cycling peptides, or using them in intervals with breaks in between, helps prevent tolerance and maintains effectiveness over time. It also gives your body a chance to recalibrate between cycles.

Typical Cycle Durations: Common cycles include 6-8 weeks of use, followed by a 2-4 week break. Adjust cycles based on the specific peptide and your body's response.

Track Progress Over Time: Document changes in energy levels, muscle tone, skin health, or other targeted benefits throughout the cycle. Use this information to determine the optimal cycle length for each peptide.

3. Monitor Health Markers Regularly

Regular health monitoring, including blood tests and physical check-ups, provides valuable feedback on how peptides are affecting your body. This is especially important for peptides that influence hormone levels, immunity, or muscle growth.

Key Markers to Monitor: Hormone levels, liver and kidney function, immune markers, and skin health are commonly affected by peptide therapy. Consult your healthcare provider to determine which markers to monitor.

Check-Up Frequency: Aim for quarterly or biannual check-ups, depending on the peptide's effects and your healthcare provider's recommendations. Adjust peptide use based on these results to maintain balance and safety.

4. Practice Proper Storage and Handling

Storing and handling peptides correctly preserves their potency and ensures safe usage. Follow supplier instructions carefully to prevent peptide degradation.

Refrigerate When Needed: Most peptides should be stored in the refrigerator. Ensure they remain in a stable environment, away from light and heat.

Avoid Contamination: Use sterile water for reconstitution and new syringes for each injection to prevent contamination and maintain the peptide's integrity.

8.2 Dosage and Stacking Guide for Easy Reference

A well-structured dosage and stacking guide can make peptide therapy more accessible and effective. Understanding optimal dosages for different peptides, along with safe stacking combinations, allows you to tailor your regimen to maximize benefits and minimize risks. Whether you're a beginner looking for foundational guidance or an experienced user seeking advanced strategies, this reference guide offers clear recommendations on dosage ranges, stacking options, and scheduling.

Understanding Dosage and Stacking in Peptide Therapy

Dosage and stacking involve not only choosing the right peptide amounts but also combining peptides in a way that enhances their effects without compromising safety. Effective dosage ensures that each peptide is delivering its intended benefits, while stacking allows you to create a synergistic effect by combining peptides with complementary functions.

Key Considerations in Dosage and Stacking:

1. Individual Goals: Tailor your dosages and stacking choices to align with specific objectives, such as muscle growth, skin health, or immune support.

2. Safety First: Start with lower dosages, especially when stacking multiple peptides, to gauge how your body responds. Gradually increase as needed, following professional guidance.

3. Timing and Frequency: Timing affects how well peptides perform, particularly those that influence sleep, energy, or growth hormone release. Sticking to a structured schedule can improve consistency in results.

Dosage Guide for Popular Peptides

Different peptides have unique effects, and their dosages vary based on factors like purpose, body weight, and individual response. Below is a dosage reference for some of the most popular peptides, broken down by category.

1. Skin Health and Anti-Aging Peptides

These peptides support skin rejuvenation, collagen production, and general anti-aging benefits, making them ideal for skincare and wellness regimens.

- **GHK-Cu (Copper Peptide)**
Dosage: 2-5 mg per week (injection) or as directed for topical application.
Frequency: Use 2-3 times per week for injections, or daily for topical application.

Timing: Ideally administered in the evening, aligning with the skin's natural repair cycle.

Cycle Length: GHK-Cu can be used continuously, but it's often cycled in 6-8 week intervals for optimal skin health.

- **Matrixyl (Palmitoyl Pentapeptide-4)**

Dosage: Use as directed in skincare formulations, typically found in concentrations of 2-3% in creams or serums.

Frequency: Daily, morning and night as part of your skincare routine.

Timing: Apply after cleansing and before moisturizer to ensure absorption.

2. Muscle Growth and Recovery Peptides

For those focused on muscle growth, recovery, or athletic performance, these peptides aid in growth hormone release and support muscle repair.

- **CJC-1295 + Ipamorelin**

Dosage: 100-200 mcg of each peptide per dose.

Frequency: 1-2 times per day, often in the evening or before sleep to maximize growth hormone release.

Timing: Administer on an empty stomach, ideally 2 hours after the last meal.

Cycle Length: Typical cycles last 6-8 weeks, with a 2-4 week break before starting again.

- **BPC-157 (Body Protective Compound)**

Dosage: 200-500 mcg per day, adjusted based on recovery needs.

Frequency: Daily, divided into 1-2 doses, especially useful after workouts or injury.

Timing: Can be taken in the morning or post-workout, depending on your recovery goals.

Cycle Length: BPC-157 is often used for 4-6 weeks, followed by a short break if needed.

3. Immune Support and Longevity Peptides

These peptides boost immune health, improve resilience, and promote cellular longevity, making them ideal for long-term wellness and anti-aging goals.

- Epitalon

Dosage: 5-10 mg per day.

Frequency: Daily, in short cycles or as recommended for anti-aging protocols.

Timing: Divide the dose into two administrations (morning and evening) for balanced effects.

Cycle Length: Commonly used in cycles of 10-20 days, repeated 2-3 times a year for longevity benefits.

- **Thymosin Alpha-1**

Dosage: 1.6 mg per dose, adjusted based on immune needs.

Frequency: 2-3 times per week, with increased frequency during periods of immune vulnerability.

Timing: Administer in the morning or as directed by a healthcare provider.

Cycle Length: Thymosin Alpha-1 is typically cycled in 4-8 week intervals.

4. Cognitive Enhancement Peptides

These peptides support cognitive health, mental clarity, and stress resilience. They are popular among individuals seeking to boost focus, memory, or mood.

- Selank

Dosage: 250-500 mcg per dose.
Frequency: 2-3 times per day, especially during periods of high cognitive demand.
Timing: Administered throughout the day, but avoid taking too close to bedtime.
Cycle Length: Selank can be used in cycles of 4-6 weeks, depending on need.

- Semax

Dosage: 250-1,000 mcg per dose, depending on tolerance.
Frequency: 1-2 times per day.
Timing: Use in the morning or before cognitively demanding activities.
Cycle Length: Semax is often cycled for 3-4 weeks, followed by a short break.

Stacking Guide for Enhanced Results

Peptide stacking refers to the practice of combining two or more peptides to create synergistic effects. Stacking can enhance results by targeting complementary pathways, especially for individuals with multiple wellness goals.

1. Stack for Skin Rejuvenation and Anti-Aging

This stack targets skin health, helping reduce wrinkles, boost collagen production, and enhance overall skin elasticity.

Recommended Stack: GHK-Cu + Matrixyl
- Dosage: 2-5 mg per week (GHK-Cu), daily topical application (Matrixyl).
- Cycle Length**: 6-8 weeks on, followed by a short break for maintenance.

2. Stack for Muscle Growth and Recovery

Ideal for athletes and fitness enthusiasts, this stack promotes muscle growth and faster recovery, supporting workouts and active lifestyles.

Recommended Stack: CJC-1295 + Ipamorelin + BPC-157
- Dosage: 100-200 mcg each (CJC-1295 and Ipamorelin), 200-500 mcg (BPC-157).
- Timing: Administer CJC-1295 and Ipamorelin at night on an empty stomach; BPC-157 can be taken post-workout.
- Cycle Length: 6-8 weeks on, 2-4 weeks off.

3. Stack for Immune Support and Longevity

This stack boosts immune resilience and may support cellular longevity, making it ideal for anti-aging protocols.

Recommended Stack: Thymosin Alpha-1 + Epitalon

- Dosage: 1.6 mg (Thymosin Alpha-1), 5-10 mg (Epitalon) per day.
- Cycle Length: 10-20 days (Epitalon), 4-8 weeks (Thymosin Alpha-1).

4. Stack for Cognitive Enhancement and Stress Relief

Targeted at those seeking mental clarity, improved focus, and stress resilience, this stack supports cognitive health during demanding periods.

Recommended Stack: Selank + Semax
- Dosage: 250-500 mcg each, administered throughout the day.
- Cycle Length: 3-4 weeks on, 1 week off for optimal results.

Practical Tips for Dosage and Stacking Safety

When incorporating peptides into your regimen, prioritizing safety in dosage and stacking is crucial for both short- and long-term results. Here are some key safety tips to consider:

1. Start with Lower Dosages When Stacking

When using multiple peptides, starting with lower dosages helps you assess how your body responds to each peptide. Gradually increasing dosages allows your body to adapt, reducing the risk of side effects.

2. Space Out Administration Times

If stacking peptides with similar effects, space out administration times to avoid overwhelming the body. For example, growth hormone-stimulating peptides like CJC-1295 and Ipamorelin are best taken together in the evening, while recovery peptides like BPC-157 may be better suited for morning or post-workout.

3. Monitor for Side Effects and Adjust Accordingly

Keep a journal to track your body's response to each peptide, especially when stacking. Document any side effects, mood changes, or physical sensations to determine if dosage adjustments are needed.

4. Follow a Structured Cycle

Cycling your peptides prevents the body from building tolerance and ensures that you're using them at their most effective dosages. Following a structured cycle (e.g., 6-8 weeks on, 2-4 weeks off) helps maintain potency and efficacy over time.

8.3 Charts and Graphs for Visualizing Your Progress

Tracking progress with peptide therapy can be challenging, especially when trying to monitor multiple aspects of health, fitness, and wellness. Visual tools like charts and graphs make it easier to record, analyze, and adjust your regimen based on observable results. By using these tools, you can track everything from muscle gain and skin improvements to cognitive changes and recovery times, helping you see the impact of your peptides over time.

Why Visualizing Progress is Essential in Peptide Therapy

Peptide therapy involves gradual changes in various areas of health and wellness, such as skin elasticity, muscle strength, and energy levels. Tracking these changes visually through charts and graphs makes it easier to see how your body is responding to different peptides and helps you identify when adjustments are needed.

Benefits of visual progress tracking include:

1. Enhanced Motivation: Visual results can keep you motivated by showing how far you've come and what improvements have been made.
2. Improved Accuracy in Adjustments: Tracking trends in dosage, effects, and symptoms helps you make precise adjustments, maximizing benefits and reducing side effects.
3. Better Understanding of Cycles and Tolerance: Visual data enables you to identify patterns in how your body responds to peptides over time, especially in cyclic regimens.
4. Objective Assessment of Efficacy: Quantifying progress through charts and graphs provides a clearer, more objective view of what's working and what needs adjustment.

Types of Charts and Graphs for Tracking Peptide Therapy Progress

Different aspects of peptide therapy may require distinct types of charts or graphs. Here are some recommended chart types, along with suggestions for what to track within each:

1. Line Charts for Tracking Changes Over Time

Line charts are excellent for tracking gradual changes, such as improvements in skin elasticity, muscle growth, or mood stability. With line charts, you can visualize trends and identify how consistent your progress has been over a given period.

Recommended Metrics:
   Skin Elasticity: Measure using a skin elasticity meter, recording data weekly or biweekly.
   Muscle Growth: Record muscle measurements or strength indicators, such as weightlifting capabilities.
   Energy Levels: Track daily energy scores, from 1 to 10, based on how you feel throughout the day.
   Mood Stability: Score mood on a scale of 1-10 daily, noting any significant fluctuations.

2. Bar Graphs for Dosage and Response Comparisons

Bar graphs are effective for comparing responses to different dosages or peptide combinations. This graph type allows you to see how varying doses affect your body, making it useful for identifying optimal dosing strategies.

Recommended Metrics:

Dosage vs. Results: Compare the efficacy of low, medium, and high doses by tracking metrics like muscle tone, sleep quality, or skin texture.

Side Effects at Different Dosages: Record side effect intensity (1-5 scale) at varying dosages to identify tolerance levels.

Peptide Stacking Efficacy: Track results when using peptides individually versus stacked, comparing the effects of different combinations.

3. Pie Charts for Side Effect Distribution

Pie charts are a simple, visual way to show the distribution of side effects or symptoms you may experience with peptide therapy. This chart type helps you quickly identify the most common side effects, guiding dosage adjustments or changes in peptides.

Recommended Metrics:

Side Effect Types: Track the occurrence of specific side effects (e.g., headache, fatigue, injection site soreness) and represent their frequency as a percentage.

Severity of Side Effects: Divide side effects into categories (mild, moderate, severe) and show the percentage breakdown for each.

4. Progression Charts for Tracking Cycles

Progression charts allow you to see how your body responds throughout different cycles of peptide therapy. By organizing data by cycle, you can evaluate if each cycle is yielding consistent results or if adjustments are necessary.

Recommended Metrics:
  Muscle Growth per Cycle: Measure changes in muscle mass or strength at the end of each cycle.
  Skin Quality per Cycle: Use metrics like skin hydration or elasticity, measured at the beginning and end of each cycle.
  Energy and Mood Consistency: Track changes in energy and mood across cycles to see if improvements are steady or vary.

Sample Chart Templates for Peptide Therapy

Creating a consistent system for recording and interpreting data requires structured chart templates. Here are some examples of chart templates that you can customize to fit your specific tracking needs.

1. Weekly Line Chart Template for Skin Elasticity and Muscle Growth

Title: Weekly Progress Chart – Skin Elasticity and Muscle Growth

Week	Skin Elasticity Score	Bicep Circumfe -rence	Leg Press Weight	Energy Level (1-10)|
1				

2				
3				
4				

Instructions: Measure skin elasticity using a meter or subjective scale weekly. Record muscle measurements and exercise weights to gauge strength gains.

2. Monthly Bar Graph Template for Dosage vs. Efficacy

Title: Monthly Dosage vs. Efficacy Comparison

Peptide	Low Dose	Medium Dose	High Dose	Optimal Score
GHK-Cu				
CJC-129 5				
BPC-157				

Instructions: Track response scores (1-10) for different doses to identify the most effective dose for each peptide.

3. Pie Chart Template for Side Effect Distribution

Title: Side Effect Distribution – Peptide

Side Effect	Occurrence	Percentage
Headache		
Fatigue		
Injection Site Soreness		
Nausea		

Instructions: Note each side effect and its frequency, then calculate the percentage for a quick overview of common side effects.

4. Cycle Progression Chart Template for Long-Term Results

Title: Cycle Progression Chart – Muscle Growth and Energy

Cycle	Muscle Mass Gain (%)	Energy Level Score (Avg)	Mood Stability Score (Avg)
1			
2			
3			

Instructions: Record end-of-cycle metrics to track progress over multiple cycles, helping assess if the therapy is yielding consistent improvements.

Interpreting Your Data for Informed Decisions

Once you've recorded your data, analyzing patterns, trends, and shifts helps you make informed decisions about dosage, peptide combinations, and cycle adjustments. Here's how to interpret the data effectively:

1. Identify Trends in Progress

Look for upward or steady trends in data points like skin elasticity, muscle growth, or energy levels, as these often indicate consistent benefits from your regimen. Downward trends or plateauing results might suggest a need for dosage adjustments or a break between cycles.

Example: If muscle growth continues to increase with each cycle, your dosage may be effective. If growth slows down, consider slightly increasing the dose or adjusting the timing.

2. Spot Dosage-Related Side Effects

Review data from bar graphs or pie charts on side effects at different dosages. Higher frequencies or severity of side effects at specific doses can indicate the need for reduction or adjustment in dosage.

Example: If higher doses of CJC-1295 are causing headaches or fatigue, consider lowering the dose to minimize side effects while retaining efficacy.

3. Evaluate Stacking Efficacy

When stacking peptides, compare progress charts to see if combining peptides is producing more substantial or faster results compared to using them individually. If stacking yields improved outcomes, it may be a preferred approach for reaching your goals.

Example: If stacking BPC-157 with Thymosin Beta-4 improves recovery times more than BPC-157 alone, this combination may be ideal for your recovery needs.

4. Use Cycle Progression to Adjust Long-Term Goals

Cycle progression charts provide insights into how effective each cycle is over the long term. If progress stalls or side effects increase with each cycle, it may indicate the need for longer breaks, different peptides, or a revised dosage.

Example: If energy levels consistently improve across cycles, your peptide regimen is likely well-suited for energy enhancement. If energy gains diminish, consult a professional to adjust your peptide choices or dosages.

Visualizing your progress through charts and graphs empowers you to take a proactive approach to peptide therapy, helping you achieve targeted results efficiently and sustainably.

Chapter 9: The Future of Anti-Aging – New Frontiers in Peptide Research

9.1 Emerging Peptides and Their Potential

As the science of peptide therapy continues to evolve, researchers are discovering new peptides with promising anti-aging properties and exploring their potential applications in areas beyond traditional skincare and wellness. From cellular regeneration and metabolic health to cognitive enhancement and immune resilience, emerging peptides hold exciting possibilities for advancing anti-aging science and expanding our understanding of human longevity.

The Importance of Emerging Peptide Research in Anti-Aging

Peptides are small but powerful molecules that interact directly with the body's cellular and biochemical processes.

238

By mimicking natural signals, peptides have the potential to promote everything from collagen synthesis and tissue repair to hormonal balance and cognitive function. This ability to influence core physiological processes positions peptides as valuable tools in the field of anti-aging, allowing scientists to target the aging process at the molecular level.

Key areas where emerging peptides may impact anti-aging research include:

1. Cellular Regeneration: Promoting cell growth, repair, and regeneration to maintain youthful tissue function.
2. Metabolic Enhancement: Supporting metabolic health by balancing insulin sensitivity, fat metabolism, and energy production.
3. Neuroprotection and Cognitive Support: Enhancing brain health, memory, and cognitive resilience as part of holistic anti-aging practices.
4. Immune Modulation: Strengthening immune function, helping the body better respond to environmental stressors and infections.

Overview of Emerging Anti-Aging Peptides

The following peptides represent some of the most exciting advancements in peptide research, each offering unique mechanisms that could transform anti-aging therapy. While some are still undergoing studies for safety and efficacy, they provide valuable insights into the future of peptide-based anti-aging treatments.

1. MOTS-c – The Mitochondrial Peptide for Metabolic Health

MOTS-c is a mitochondrial-derived peptide that has gained attention for its potential role in enhancing metabolism, energy production, and cellular resilience. By targeting mitochondrial function, MOTS-c may help slow down age-related metabolic decline, making it a promising candidate for anti-aging therapies.

Potential Benefits:
Enhances Metabolic Health: Improves insulin sensitivity, supports fat metabolism, and reduces risk factors associated with metabolic disorders.

Boosts Cellular Energy: Increases cellular energy production, promoting vitality and resilience to stress.

Protects Against Age-Related Diseases: Preliminary research suggests MOTS-c may help mitigate age-related diseases by supporting mitochondrial health.

Current Research: Studies on MOTS-c are exploring its applications in metabolic syndrome, obesity, and insulin resistance. While still in the experimental phase, MOTS-c holds potential as a therapeutic agent for metabolic and age-related conditions.

2. FOXO4-DRI – Targeting Senescent Cells for Longevity

FOXO4-DRI is an innovative peptide designed to address cellular senescence, a process where cells lose the ability to divide and function, leading to tissue aging and age-related diseases. By selectively targeting and clearing senescent cells, FOXO4-DRI could reduce inflammation and promote healthier cellular environments.

Potential Benefits:

Reduces Senescent Cells: Helps remove dysfunctional cells from the body, reducing inflammation and improving tissue health.

Enhances Longevity: May slow the aging process by improving cellular turnover and maintaining tissue integrity.

Supports Organ Function: Potential to improve overall organ health and resilience to age-related damage.

Current Research: FOXO4-DRI is in preclinical research, with studies showing promising results in animal models. As research progresses, it may become a core component of anti-aging protocols focused on cellular rejuvenation.

3. Thymulin – Immunomodulatory Peptide for Immune Support

Thymulin, a thymic peptide hormone, plays a crucial role in immune function, specifically in the development and regulation of T-cells. Its potential in anti-aging lies in its ability to restore youthful immune function, making it particularly relevant for older individuals or those with compromised immunity.

Potential Benefits:

Boosts Immune Resilience: Supports immune cell production and helps maintain a balanced immune response.

Reduces Inflammatory Markers: May lower chronic inflammation, a common contributor to aging and age-related diseases.

Enhances Immune Health in Aging Populations: Helps counteract the natural decline in immune function associated with aging.

Current Research: Studies are ongoing to explore Thymulin's effects on age-related immune decline and autoimmune conditions. Researchers are optimistic about its role in immune modulation and chronic disease prevention.

4. DSIP (Delta Sleep-Inducing Peptide) – Enhancing Restorative Sleep

Quality sleep is crucial for physical and mental well-being, yet it often declines with age. DSIP is a peptide that has shown potential in promoting deep, restorative sleep, making it valuable for anti-aging therapies focused on sleep improvement.

Potential Benefits:
Improves Sleep Quality: Promotes deep sleep stages, supporting mental clarity, physical recovery, and emotional resilience.

Reduces Stress and Fatigue: Alleviates stress-related insomnia, helping improve sleep consistency.

Supports Cognitive Function: Improved sleep quality has a positive impact on memory, focus, and overall cognitive health.

Current Research: DSIP is being studied for its sleep-regulating properties, with initial findings showing promise in sleep disorders and stress-related conditions. Its application in anti-aging therapies may help address sleep disturbances common in older adults.

5. PNC-27 – A Potential Anti-Cancer Peptide

PNC-27 is a peptide developed with a unique focus: selectively targeting cancer cells. Although still in its early stages of research, PNC-27 has shown potential for selectively binding to and eliminating cancer cells, making it a peptide with potential implications for cancer prevention and treatment.

Potential Benefits:
  Selective Targeting of Cancer Cells: PNC-27 appears to differentiate between healthy and cancerous cells, offering a targeted approach.
  Reduces Cancer Growth: Early research suggests PNC-27 may inhibit cancer cell proliferation, though more studies are needed.
  Potential for Cancer Prevention: As an emerging therapy, PNC-27 could become a preventive measure against certain cancers in high-risk individuals.

Current Research: Studies are focused on its mechanism of action and potential applications in oncology. While much remains to be explored, the peptide's unique targeting capability makes it a candidate for future anti-aging therapies that emphasize cancer prevention.

6. AOD9604 – Fat Loss and Metabolic Support

AOD9604 is a modified form of the human growth hormone fragment, developed specifically for fat loss and metabolic enhancement. Unlike traditional growth hormone, AOD9604 focuses on fat metabolism without affecting muscle growth or causing unwanted side effects.

Potential Benefits:
 Promotes Fat Reduction: Supports lipolysis (fat breakdown), aiding in fat loss while preserving lean muscle.

Improves Metabolic Health: May boost energy levels and support healthy metabolic function, especially beneficial in aging individuals.

Non-Stimulant Fat Loss: Provides a fat-reducing effect without the stimulant-like effects of other weight-loss methods.

Current Research: AOD9604 is undergoing studies for its safety profile and potential as a therapeutic for obesity and metabolic disorders. Its targeted fat loss properties make it a valuable candidate for anti-aging protocols focused on body composition.

7. Humanin – Mitochondrial Peptide for Cellular Protection

Humanin is another mitochondrial-derived peptide, similar to MOTS-c, with a focus on cellular protection and metabolic regulation. It has shown promise in protecting against oxidative stress, which is a key factor in cellular aging.

Potential Benefits:

Protects Against Oxidative Stress: Reduces cell damage from free radicals, supporting longevity and cellular health.

Promotes Energy Efficiency: Enhances mitochondrial function, increasing cellular energy production.

Supports Brain Health: May reduce the risk of neurodegenerative conditions by protecting neurons from age-related damage.

Current Research: Humanin is being explored for its neuroprotective and metabolic benefits, with potential applications in age-related diseases such as Alzheimer's and metabolic syndrome. As research advances, Humanin may play a role in comprehensive anti-aging strategies.

Emerging Peptides: Challenges and Future Directions

While the potential of these emerging peptides is exciting, several challenges remain before they can become mainstream anti-aging therapies. Ongoing research, clinical trials, and regulatory approval are essential to ensure safety and efficacy. Key areas of focus for future research include:

- Long-Term Safety Studies: Understanding the long-term effects of emerging peptides, especially those that affect cellular metabolism or immune function, is crucial for safe use in anti-aging.
- Refining Dosage and Delivery: Determining optimal dosages, delivery methods, and timing can improve peptide efficacy and minimize side effects.

- Broadening Accessibility: As research progresses, making these peptides widely available and affordable will be essential for integrating them into anti-aging practices.
- Ethics and Regulation: Regulatory bodies are carefully monitoring peptide therapies to ensure they are safe, effective, and ethically produced, particularly for peptides with therapeutic implications like PNC-27.

The Potential Impact of Emerging Peptides on Anti-Aging

As peptide research advances, we may see a new era in anti-aging that focuses on prevention, cellular rejuvenation, and metabolic health. These emerging peptides offer tools to address age-related decline from multiple angles, providing a more holistic approach to maintaining youthfulness and resilience. With continued research, we may soon access peptide therapies capable of delaying, or even reversing, aspects of the aging process.

9.2 Innovations in Anti-Aging and Biohacking

As science and technology continue to push the boundaries of anti-aging, new methods and practices are emerging that allow individuals to take control of their health, wellness, and longevity like never before. This era of *biohacking*—the use of science and technology to optimize physical and mental health—intersects with anti-aging research in fascinating ways. By understanding how biohacking and anti-aging innovations complement each other, we can explore exciting new frontiers in sustaining youth, vitality, and wellness for longer.

Biohacking and Anti-Aging: A Powerful Partnership

Biohacking has evolved from simple lifestyle adjustments to complex, data-driven practices that target the very roots of aging. By combining biohacking techniques with scientific advancements in anti-aging, individuals can address aging at multiple levels, from cellular health to brain function. Areas where biohacking aligns with anti-aging include:

1. Genetic and Epigenetic Modulation: Targeting the genes and epigenetic markers that influence aging can lead to more personalized anti-aging strategies.
2. Metabolic and Hormonal Optimization: Biohackers focus on balancing metabolism and hormones to prevent age-related metabolic decline.
3. Enhanced Physical and Cognitive Function: Biohacking practices can optimize physical resilience and cognitive sharpness, extending vitality well into later life.

Innovative Technologies in Anti-Aging and Biohacking

Recent technological advancements are reshaping anti-aging practices by providing more precise, personalized, and effective ways to slow down or even reverse aspects of aging.

1. Advanced Diagnostic Tools

Precision diagnostics allow individuals to understand their unique biological makeup, making it possible to tailor anti-aging practices more effectively. These tools provide insights into genetic predispositions, biological age, hormone levels, and cellular health, offering a roadmap for personalized anti-aging interventions.

Genetic Testing and Analysis: Advanced genetic testing can reveal predispositions to certain age-related conditions, allowing for preventive measures. Tests like 23andMe or more specialized anti-aging panels can identify genes associated with metabolism, skin health, cognitive function, and other key areas.

Biological Age Measurement: Tools that measure biological age, as opposed to chronological age, provide a realistic picture of how quickly the body is aging. Biological age tests, which often assess DNA methylation patterns, allow users to track the effectiveness of anti-aging interventions over time.

Metabolic and Hormonal Profiling: Comprehensive blood panels and hormone assessments allow biohackers to optimize their metabolism and hormonal balance, which are crucial for sustained energy and physical resilience as they age.

2. Peptide Therapy for Targeted Anti-Aging Effects

Peptide therapy is one of the most exciting innovations in anti-aging and biohacking, allowing for targeted interventions in skin health, muscle growth, immune function, and cellular regeneration. With advancements in peptide formulation and delivery, biohackers can now use peptides more effectively and safely.

Customized Peptide Stacking: With more knowledge of peptide interactions, individuals can now design custom stacks that target multiple aging aspects at once. For example, combining peptides that enhance sleep quality (like DSIP) with those that promote cellular regeneration (like MOTS-c) can create a synergistic anti-aging effect.

Precision Dosage and Delivery: Innovations in peptide delivery, such as microneedle patches and controlled-release injections, enable precise dosing, maximizing therapeutic effects while minimizing potential side effects.

Cellular Regeneration and Repair: Peptides like Epitalon and FOXO4-DRI specifically target cellular health, promoting longevity and protecting against age-related decline.

3. Genetic and Epigenetic Biohacking

Genetic and epigenetic biohacking targets the very core of the aging process. By manipulating how genes are expressed or editing genetic material, biohackers are now exploring ways to slow or even reverse cellular aging.

CRISPR Gene Editing: CRISPR (Clustered Regularly Interspaced Short Palindromic Repeats) allows scientists to edit DNA sequences directly, making it a powerful tool for correcting genetic mutations associated with aging. While CRISPR is primarily used in research settings, the technology holds promise for future anti-aging applications.

Epigenetic Reprogramming: Epigenetic modifications, such as DNA methylation and histone modification, influence gene expression without altering the underlying genetic code.

Biohackers use dietary adjustments, supplements, and specific exercise regimens to encourage favorable epigenetic changes that support longevity and vitality.

Senolytics: Senolytic compounds are designed to selectively target and remove senescent cells, which are dysfunctional cells that accumulate with age and contribute to inflammation. By reducing senescent cell load, senolytics may improve tissue health and potentially extend lifespan.

Biohacking Strategies for Anti-Aging

Beyond advanced technology and therapy, biohackers are embracing lifestyle practices and supplements that help counteract the effects of aging. These practices often focus on optimizing cellular function, improving cognitive resilience, and sustaining physical performance.

1. Nutritional Biohacking

Nutrition plays a pivotal role in anti-aging, as the foods and supplements consumed directly impact cellular health, inflammation, and metabolic function. Biohackers focus on dietary strategies that promote longevity and enhance overall wellness.

Intermittent Fasting and Caloric Restriction: Intermittent fasting (IF) and caloric restriction (CR) have been shown to improve metabolic health, reduce oxidative stress, and extend lifespan in animal studies. IF and CR encourage autophagy, a cellular cleanup process that removes damaged components and supports regeneration.

Antioxidant-Rich Diets: Diets high in antioxidants from sources like berries, dark leafy greens, and nuts help reduce oxidative damage, one of the primary contributors to aging.

NAD+ Precursors: Nicotinamide adenine dinucleotide (NAD+) is a molecule that supports cellular energy production and DNA repair. Supplements like NMN (nicotinamide mononucleotide) and NR (nicotinamide riboside) boost NAD+ levels, promoting cellular repair and potentially extending lifespan.

2. Hormone Optimization

As people age, hormone levels naturally decline, affecting energy, muscle mass, cognitive function, and mood. Biohackers aim to maintain balanced hormone levels to counteract these effects and promote vitality.

Testosterone and Estrogen Modulation: For men, testosterone replacement therapy (TRT) can improve muscle mass, energy levels, and cognitive function. For women, bioidentical hormone replacement therapy (BHRT) can balance estrogen and progesterone, supporting skin health, mood stability, and bone density.

Human Growth Hormone (HGH) and IGF-1: Growth hormone levels decline with age, leading to muscle loss and reduced metabolic function. Peptide-based therapies, such as Ipamorelin, stimulate natural HGH release, providing benefits without the downsides of synthetic HGH.

Thyroid Support: Optimizing thyroid hormone levels ensures efficient metabolism and energy production. Biohackers often monitor thyroid function and supplement with compounds that support thyroid health, like iodine and selenium.

3. Cognitive Enhancement and Neuroprotection

Biohacking practices aimed at cognitive health focus on improving memory, focus, and emotional resilience. As cognitive function naturally declines with age, enhancing brain health is essential for maintaining quality of life.

Nootropic Stacks: Nootropics are supplements that support cognitive function. Biohackers use natural and synthetic nootropics like L-theanine, caffeine, and racetams to improve memory, attention, and mood.
Brain-Derived Neurotrophic Factor (BDNF): BDNF is a protein that promotes neuron growth and resilience. Exercise, intermittent fasting, and supplements like omega-3s are known to boost BDNF levels, enhancing brain health and cognitive function.
Neuroprotective Peptides: Peptides like Selank and Semax are used to support cognitive health, especially during periods of high stress or mental demand, by reducing anxiety and promoting focus.

Future Directions in Anti-Aging and Biohacking

The combination of biohacking and anti-aging innovations opens up new possibilities for wellness and longevity. Research and development are likely to focus on making these advancements more accessible, affordable, and effective for the general population.

1. Personalized Medicine and Artificial Intelligence (AI)

As data collection and analysis improve, artificial intelligence will play an increasing role in personalizing anti-aging treatments. AI can process large amounts of data, enabling healthcare providers to tailor recommendations for everything from peptide therapies to dietary plans.

Customized Peptide Regimens: AI-powered algorithms could design optimal peptide stacks based on individual genetic and metabolic profiles, maximizing effectiveness and minimizing side effects.
Predictive Aging Models: Machine learning models can predict how a person's lifestyle choices and genetic factors influence their biological age, allowing for preventive adjustments.
Smart Diagnostic Tools: Wearable technology integrated with AI can continuously monitor biomarkers like heart rate, glucose levels, and stress markers, providing real-time insights into health status and early detection of age-related changes.

2. Regenerative Medicine and Stem Cell Therapy

Stem cell therapy and regenerative medicine offer powerful anti-aging potential, as they promote tissue repair, immune support, and cellular regeneration.

Mesenchymal Stem Cells (MSCs): MSCs are being used in research to rejuvenate aging tissues, reduce inflammation, and support immune health. Stem cell therapy holds promise for treating conditions associated with aging, like arthritis, neurodegeneration, and cardiovascular disease.

Induced Pluripotent Stem Cells (iPSCs): iPSCs are stem cells that can differentiate into any cell type, making them valuable for regenerative medicine. Researchers are exploring ways to use iPSCs to repair damaged organs, improve skin health, and enhance tissue resilience.

Exosome Therapy: Exosomes, which are small vesicles released by cells, carry bioactive molecules that support cell communication and tissue repair. Exosome therapy is an emerging field that could promote healing and reduce inflammation in aging tissues.

3. Augmented Reality (AR) and Virtual Reality (VR) for Mental and Physical Wellness

Augmented reality and virtual reality have applications beyond entertainment; they are being developed as therapeutic tools for physical and cognitive health.

VR Fitness and Rehabilitation: Virtual reality is used to create engaging exercise routines that encourage physical activity and improve motor skills, helping individuals maintain muscle tone, flexibility, and coordination.

AR Cognitive Training: Augmented reality tools offer cognitive exercises that enhance memory, focus, and problem-solving skills, benefiting mental agility.

Mental Health Applications: VR experiences can create calming environments that support meditation, stress reduction, and mental clarity, contributing to emotional wellness.

The marriage of biohacking and anti-aging innovation is paving the way for a future where age becomes just a number, and health can be actively preserved and optimized across a lifetime.

9.3 A Look Ahead: How Peptides Are Shaping the Future of Youth and Wellness

Peptides, once the domain of specialized medical treatments and niche research, are fast becoming central to the pursuit of wellness and youthfulness in a way that could fundamentally change how we approach aging. With ongoing advancements in peptide science, these tiny chains of amino acids are being tailored to address age-related challenges with unprecedented precision. As more individuals seek ways to age gracefully and maintain health across their lives, peptides are emerging as some of the most promising tools available.

The Vision for Peptides in Anti-Aging and Youthful Wellness

Peptides offer a unique advantage in anti-aging because they work at the cellular level, where aging processes originate. Unlike traditional approaches that focus on treating symptoms or external signs of aging, peptides address the root causes, such as cellular damage, metabolic decline, and hormonal shifts. By directly influencing these fundamental processes, peptides can promote regeneration, enhance immune function, improve cognitive resilience, and support other aspects of health that typically decline with age.

The future of peptides in wellness and anti-aging is characterized by:

1. Personalized Medicine: Customizing peptide therapies to each individual's unique genetic, metabolic, and lifestyle factors.
2. Comprehensive Anti-Aging Strategies: Integrating peptides with lifestyle interventions for a holistic approach to longevity.
3. Preventive Health: Using peptides not just to address aging symptoms but to delay or prevent age-related diseases.

Emerging Peptide Applications: Addressing Aging Beyond Skin and Muscle

While peptides like GHK-Cu and CJC-1295 have demonstrated remarkable efficacy in skin and muscle health, research is revealing applications far beyond these areas. Next-generation peptides are now being developed to target specific age-related processes that go beyond aesthetics or fitness.

1. Peptides for Cognitive Resilience

Age-related cognitive decline remains one of the most challenging aspects of aging, affecting quality of life and independence. Future peptide therapies may address these cognitive challenges by enhancing brain health, supporting memory formation, and promoting neuroprotection.

Potential Peptides:

Dihexa: A promising peptide known to promote synaptogenesis (the formation of connections between neurons), Dihexa may enhance memory and cognitive function.

Cerebrolysin: This peptide mix supports neuroplasticity and brain resilience, and early research suggests it may aid in neuroprotection for aging populations.

Humanin: Already known for its mitochondrial benefits, Humanin also has neuroprotective properties that could reduce the risk of neurodegenerative conditions.

2. Peptides for Metabolic Health and Weight Management

Maintaining a healthy metabolism is essential for longevity, as it influences energy levels, body composition, and disease risk. Peptides that target metabolic health are being designed to promote fat loss, improve insulin sensitivity, and prevent metabolic disorders.

Potential Peptides:

MOTS-c: This mitochondrial peptide supports cellular energy and insulin sensitivity, helping combat age-related metabolic slowdown.

AOD9604: A modified growth hormone fragment focused on fat metabolism, AOD9604 aids in reducing body fat while preserving muscle mass.

Tirzepatide: Originally designed to manage blood sugar, tirzepatide has shown potential in promoting weight loss, making it valuable for metabolic health.

3. Peptides for Immune System Support

Aging is often associated with a decline in immune function, leading to increased vulnerability to infections and chronic inflammation. Peptides that strengthen the immune system can support the body's natural defenses, potentially lowering the risk of age-related illnesses.

Potential Peptides:
Thymosin Alpha-1: Known for its immune-modulating properties, Thymosin Alpha-1 promotes T-cell production and is being studied for its potential to counteract immune aging.
Thymosin Beta-4: This peptide aids in tissue repair and reduces inflammation, supporting immune resilience and recovery.
Epitalon: Beyond its effects on telomeres, Epitalon may enhance the immune system by promoting thymus gland health.

Integrating Peptides with Modern Lifestyle Choices for Enhanced Youthfulness

As peptides continue to evolve, their effectiveness will be maximized by integrating them with complementary lifestyle choices. This means that the future of anti-aging peptides will likely involve a combination of personalized peptide therapy, nutrition, exercise, and biohacking strategies, creating a comprehensive approach to wellness.

1. Nutrition and Supplement Synergy

Peptides and nutrition work together to support cellular health and regenerative processes. Certain nutrients, like amino acids, vitamins, and antioxidants, enhance peptide activity, allowing individuals to tailor their diet to maximize anti-aging benefits.

Essential Nutrients: Amino acids (like glycine, glutamine, and arginine) support peptide synthesis and cellular repair. Omega-3 fatty acids and vitamins C and E are also crucial for reducing inflammation and oxidative stress.
NAD+ Precursors: Nicotinamide riboside (NR) and nicotinamide mononucleotide (NMN) are supplements that boost NAD+ levels, supporting energy production, cellular repair, and the effectiveness of anti-aging peptides like Epitalon.
Intermittent Fasting: Caloric restriction and intermittent fasting activate autophagy, a cellular process that removes damaged components and promotes longevity. Combined with peptides like MOTS-c, fasting can enhance metabolic and cellular benefits.

2. Exercise and Physical Activity

Exercise is a cornerstone of healthy aging, and combining physical activity with peptide therapy can enhance both muscle resilience and cardiovascular health. Peptides that support growth hormone release, recovery, and fat metabolism align well with exercise routines.

Resistance Training and Peptides for Muscle Growth: Peptides like CJC-1295 and Ipamorelin can amplify the effects of strength training by promoting muscle recovery and hypertrophy.
Cardiovascular Health and Metabolic Peptides: Endurance exercises like running or cycling, when paired with metabolic peptides like MOTS-c, improve cardiovascular fitness and metabolic resilience.
Joint and Tissue Support: Recovery-focused peptides such as BPC-157 and Thymosin Beta-4 can support active lifestyles, reducing injury risk and speeding up recovery times.

3. Mindfulness and Stress Management

Chronic stress accelerates aging by increasing inflammation and oxidative damage. Future anti-aging practices will likely incorporate peptides that help manage stress, enhance sleep, and promote mental clarity, in addition to lifestyle changes.

Sleep-Enhancing Peptides: Peptides like DSIP (Delta Sleep-Inducing Peptide) encourage restful sleep, supporting immune resilience, cognitive function, and overall energy levels.
Mood and Cognitive Peptides: Neuropeptides such as Selank and Semax can improve focus, reduce anxiety, and protect brain health, particularly during high-stress periods.
Mindfulness Practices: Techniques such as meditation, deep breathing, and relaxation exercises enhance the effects of

anti-aging peptides by reducing cortisol levels and promoting cellular repair.

Future Directions: The Role of Peptides in Preventive Medicine

Peptides are poised to play an increasingly important role in preventive medicine, shifting the focus from treating diseases to preventing them before they arise. This shift aligns with the growing emphasis on longevity, where the goal is not just to extend life span but to enhance health span—the period during which individuals remain active and free from disease.

1. Telomere Maintenance and Cellular Longevity

Telomeres, the protective caps on chromosomes, shorten with each cell division, eventually leading to cellular aging. Peptides like Epitalon that support telomere length are gaining attention for their potential to slow this process.

Potential Benefits:
Extended Cellular Health: By maintaining telomere length, Epitalon and similar peptides may keep cells functioning optimally for longer.
Reduced Risk of Age-Related Diseases: Telomere preservation is associated with lower risks of conditions like cardiovascular disease, diabetes, and neurodegenerative disorders.

2. Addressing Inflammation and Oxidative Stress

Chronic inflammation and oxidative stress are major contributors to aging, linked to everything from cardiovascular disease to cancer. Future peptide therapies will likely focus on controlling inflammation and reducing oxidative damage to promote longevity.

Inflammation-Reducing Peptides: Peptides like Thymosin Beta-4 and BPC-157 have anti-inflammatory properties that may help manage chronic inflammation, a core factor in aging.
Antioxidant Peptides: Some peptides can stimulate the body's natural antioxidant defenses, protecting cells from oxidative damage and improving overall cellular health.

3. Early Disease Detection and Intervention

Advancements in diagnostic tools are making it possible to detect diseases earlier, allowing for peptide-based interventions that could prevent conditions from developing fully. By monitoring biomarkers and identifying early signs of aging-related changes, individuals can take proactive steps to preserve health.

Biomarker Tracking: Monitoring biomarkers like inflammatory markers, metabolic indicators, and hormone levels can help tailor peptide therapies to individual needs.
Preventive Peptide Protocols: Future peptide therapies may be designed as preventive protocols, with individuals starting peptides before symptoms of age-related conditions appear, providing a proactive approach to wellness.

As we look to the future, peptides hold the potential to redefine aging, offering tools to stay healthy, active, and mentally sharp well into our later years. By embracing these advancements, the next generation of anti-aging practices promises a future where wellness and vitality are within reach at any age.

Conclusion: Embracing a Lifelong Anti-Aging Journey

Aging is a journey, one that brings a wealth of experiences, wisdom, and personal growth. Yet as we gain years, it's natural to want to sustain the vitality, health, and strength that fuel our quality of life. Advances in science and a deeper understanding of human biology have opened a new world of possibilities, allowing us to proactively support our bodies and minds as we age. Peptide therapy, combined with holistic wellness practices, offers a powerful means to not just address the signs of aging but to embrace it as a journey marked by empowerment, resilience, and intentional living.

Reframing Aging: From Challenge to Opportunity

Historically, aging has often been viewed as an inevitable decline, marked by reduced energy, physical limitations, and cognitive slowing. However, a shift is underway—a shift from seeing aging as an inevitable set of limitations to viewing it as a stage of life that can be actively supported. This new perspective, fueled by scientific advancements, empowers individuals to take control of their aging process through intentional lifestyle choices, preventive measures, and, increasingly, innovations like peptide therapy.

Key aspects of this reframing include:

1. Focus on Health Span Over Life Span: While extending life span is important, a growing emphasis on health span—the years spent in good health, free from disease or disability—has changed the goals of anti-aging strategies. The aim is not merely to live longer but to live better, remaining active, independent, and fulfilled.

2. Holistic Approach: Anti-aging is more than skin deep; it involves every system in the body, from physical endurance and mental clarity to emotional resilience and immune strength. This holistic approach acknowledges that the entire body works in harmony and that no single solution can sustain youth on its own.

3. Proactive, Preventive Mindset: Rather than waiting until the effects of aging are deeply felt, today's anti-aging strategies encourage proactive, preventive measures that strengthen the body and mind long before signs of decline appear.

Embracing Peptide Therapy as Part of Lifelong Wellness

Peptides represent a significant advancement in the anti-aging field, allowing targeted support for specific areas of health—whether it's improving skin elasticity, enhancing muscle tone, supporting cognitive health, or boosting immune function. Integrating peptide therapy into a lifelong wellness routine provides an adaptable, evidence-based method to maintain vitality across the aging process.

The Role of Peptides in Lifelong Health

Peptides offer a way to tailor support to specific aging concerns, making them a valuable component of a comprehensive anti-aging routine:

Skin and Connective Tissue: With peptides like GHK-Cu, it's possible to directly support skin health, collagen production, and wound healing, sustaining the skin's natural resilience over time.

Muscle and Bone Health: Growth hormone-releasing peptides like CJC-1295 and Ipamorelin help support muscle growth, improve recovery, and maintain bone density, all of which are crucial for staying physically active and mobile.

Cognitive and Emotional Wellbeing: Peptides like Selank and Semax can offer neuroprotective benefits and help mitigate age-related cognitive changes, enhancing memory, focus, and emotional stability.

Immune Function and Inflammation: Peptides such as Thymosin Alpha-1 help bolster the immune system, making the body more resilient to age-related immune decline and inflammation.

These targeted effects make peptides a versatile, adaptable tool that can evolve alongside individual needs, from maintaining muscle tone in middle age to supporting cognitive health and immune function in later years.

Building a Supportive Anti-Aging Lifestyle

While peptides offer substantial benefits, it's important to recognize that they are most effective when combined with a supportive lifestyle. Aging gracefully involves a synergy of practices that create a foundation of wellness, empowering individuals to live each phase of life with confidence and vitality.

1. Nutrition as a Cornerstone of Longevity

Nutrition is one of the most powerful tools we have to influence health and aging. A diet rich in antioxidants, healthy fats, lean proteins, and complex carbohydrates fuels the body, protects against oxidative damage, and supports cellular health. Incorporating nutrient-dense foods like berries, leafy greens, nuts, and seeds can improve energy levels, support cognitive function, and enhance overall resilience to aging.

Whole-Foods-Based Diet: Emphasizing whole, unprocessed foods reduces the intake of artificial additives and refined sugars, both of which can contribute to inflammation and oxidative stress.
Intermittent Fasting: This eating pattern has been shown to promote cellular cleanup (autophagy), which can reduce cellular damage and enhance metabolic efficiency, particularly when combined with peptides like MOTS-c that support mitochondrial health.
Hydration and Skin Health: Staying well-hydrated is essential for maintaining skin elasticity and function. Drinking water, supplemented with electrolytes, helps to maintain moisture balance and nutrient transport, crucial for anti-aging efforts.

2. Physical Activity for Strength and Resilience

Exercise is foundational to aging well, offering physical, mental, and emotional benefits. Strength training, aerobic exercises, flexibility routines, and balance-focused movements help maintain muscle mass, cardiovascular health, and bone density. Regular physical activity also boosts mood, reduces the risk of chronic diseases, and even supports cognitive function.

Resistance Training: Building and maintaining muscle mass is critical for metabolic health, physical strength, and joint support. Combining exercise with peptides like CJC-1295 enhances muscle growth and recovery, making it easier to stay active and resilient as you age.

Flexibility and Mobility Exercises: Stretching, yoga, and other forms of flexibility training keep joints limber, reduce the risk of injury, and maintain range of motion, which is particularly valuable in later life.

Endurance Activities: Cardiovascular exercises like brisk walking, cycling, and swimming promote heart health, circulation, and energy levels, supporting both physical and cognitive longevity.

3. Cognitive Health and Stress Management

Aging gracefully includes nurturing mental and emotional resilience. As stress and cognitive decline can accelerate aging, prioritizing mental health is essential for a balanced anti-aging journey.

Mindfulness Practices: Meditation, deep breathing, and yoga foster emotional balance, reduce stress, and support cognitive health, complementing peptides like Selank that provide neuroprotective benefits.

Lifelong Learning: Engaging in mentally stimulating activities, such as reading, learning new skills, or solving puzzles, keeps the brain active and supports neuroplasticity, reducing the risk of cognitive decline.

Quality Sleep: Sleep is essential for physical and mental restoration. Peptides like DSIP can aid in promoting deeper, more restorative sleep, while practices like sleep hygiene, regular sleep schedules, and stress management support restful sleep naturally.

4. Regular Health Monitoring and Preventive Care

One of the most empowering aspects of a lifelong anti-aging journey is the ability to proactively monitor health. Routine health check-ups, diagnostic tests, and screenings help catch potential issues early, allowing for preventive measures and early intervention.

Annual Health Check-Ups: Regular health screenings, including blood pressure, blood sugar, cholesterol, and other markers, provide insights into overall health and help identify areas for improvement.

Biomarker Tracking: With the growing availability of wearable devices and home tests, it's easier to track markers like heart rate, sleep quality, stress levels, and even certain genetic predispositions, empowering individuals to make informed health decisions.

Genetic Testing and Personalized Medicine: Genetic testing enables a personalized approach to anti-aging, allowing individuals to understand their unique risks and optimize peptide therapy, diet, and lifestyle based on their genetic profile.

Embracing Aging with Confidence and Joy

Ultimately, the goal of a lifelong anti-aging journey isn't to deny aging but to navigate it with confidence, purpose, and joy. Aging is a natural process, but how we experience it is largely within our control. By taking a proactive, holistic approach to health, we can maximize our quality of life, enjoy vitality at every stage, and continue pursuing our passions, relationships, and personal growth without constraint. Embracing aging involves:

A Positive Mindset: Viewing aging as an opportunity for growth, exploration, and continued learning can transform how we experience this stage of life.

Adapting Goals: Recognizing that health goals evolve allows us to stay engaged and motivated as we age. What we prioritize in our 40s may differ from our goals in our 70s, but each phase is an opportunity for personal growth.

Celebrating Small Wins: From maintaining muscle strength to achieving restful sleep, celebrating each milestone creates a rewarding journey that reinforces our commitment to health and wellness.

A lifelong anti-aging journey is an investment in ourselves, allowing us to live fully and purposefully through every stage of life. With the tools and knowledge available today, each of us has the power to shape our health journey, embracing aging with confidence and celebrating the unique richness that each year brings.

www.ingramcontent.com/pod-product-compliance
Lightning Source LLC
Chambersburg PA
CBHW081545250726

48653CB00009B/3283